Finding Healing
in God's
Backyard

(STUDENT EDITION: VOLUME ONE)

Jessica Linhart

ISBN 978-1-63575-118-5 (Paperback)
ISBN 978-1-63575-119-2 (Digital)

Christian Faith Publishing, Inc.
296 Chestnut Street
Meadville, PA 16335
www.christianfaithpublishing.com

Printed in the United States of America

Acknowledgments

I would like to thank a number of people who have taught classes and gave sermons I attended. They truly provided wisdom and knowledge through their faith and instructions from God. I would like to thank my teachers: Debbie Ferrell, Donna Short, Katie Marr, Travis Asbury, and Dennis Thaxton. I would also like to share my gratitude to my preachers, Christopher Sizemore, Steven Samples, Gene Sowards, Steve Sampson, and J. J. Layne. Furthermore, I would like to give a special thank-you to my Bible study buddies: Bernie Carper, Lori Selbe Rice, Karen Taylor, David Daniels, Sandee Gilmore, Alice Robinson, Jessica Mcgraw, Brenda Ferrell, Dorinda Hudson, and Becky Moore Stinson.

Contents

Why?

This book is intended for everyone who is interested in discovering essential oils. The objective of this volume is anticipated to enhance your analysis of God's Word. This reading focuses on essential oils and also investigates the Holy Scriptures. The student edition is assembled for effortless usage. First, the information is conveyed in a question-answer format followed by scriptural opportunities. During the scriptural opportunities (homework), you will be asked to record the scriptures. This book is filled with graphic organizers to help manage your thoughts. Also included in this book are sample recipes and essential oil projects. All the assignments will help you connect to the Bible. Also, the Bible is God's attempt to create a conversation with his people. This is why we need to read and study it. Through the use of this study, you will be able to foster your relationship with Christ. Beginning with the next section, the author has provided you with space to record the scripture and to take notes.

The mission of this manuscript is to be a teaching and learning instrument. For example, essential oils are natural oils that are typically obtained by distillation. Essential oils have characteristics of fragrance found in multiple plant resins and gums. In addition, through the scriptures, we will discover how God established special plants, resins, and gums just for all mankind (Gen. 1: 11–12). God ordained vegetation and the use of natural oils in his Holy Word. Come, let us discover how we can use God's Word to explain how his creation can expand our minds, bodies, and souls (Matt. 28:19).

This book is not intended to make medical claims. The book does not suggest you create a new medication and treat yourself. Through reading this book, reading God's Word, and studying from other sources, you will develop the knowledge of how people in biblical times depended on essential oils to flourish in their daily lives. Next, you will encounter the way our society incorporates essential oils. Our society uses applications of the essential oils to enhance our lives. Furthermore, this book does not encourage anyone to prescribe or diagnose a medical condition. This manuscript recommends that you consult your physicians and medical facilities for medical care.

Additionally, this book was created in obedience to the Lord (Acts 5:29). The commitment of this project is to educate the public on the topic of essential oils. The expectation of this research is that it will provide the church with an informative Bible study, direct sales companies with a complete guide for hosting successful classes, and perhaps develop a great program for private schools. When you have completed this book, it will become a study guide for those who wish to take the opportunity to become closer to Jesus. Finally, may this book be used as a method others can use to teach and spread the Gospel.

Throughout this edition of the book, scriptures are referenced. The author has included space to record the scriptures. Educational experts state that if we write something down, we are 40 percent more likely to remember the information.

Testimony

My life, like many, is very twisted! I grew up with an empty pocketbook but with a loving family. God was there every step of the way. Yes, even in times we were not looking for him, he took care of us (Isa. 40:10).

_____

_____

_____

Jesus loves the outcasts. The poor folks hold a special place in his heart (James 2:5).

_____

_____

_____

God helped me through school, college, graduate school, marriage, and now in my current place. Just a few years ago (2007), I went into the hospital; they found postural orthostatic tachycardia syndrome (POTS), blood clots, a brain aneurysm, and a few more conditions. When we tried to repair the aneurysm, it caused too many mini-strokes to count, but Thank God, it did not take the vision of my left eye. At that moment, the mini-strokes left my body in a wrinkled-up state. Also, on the left side of my body, I had no feeling and had very little movement because that side was so stiff and heavy. My face was impaired and my speech was slurred. My memory was erased! I repented of my sin, and Jesus brought me victory—just like the old hymn states. Currently, I'm left with five mesh coils behind my right eye.

With my mother praying by my side every day and God's elect praying, God healed my body, my soul, and my mind. He created a new creature in me (2 Cor. 2:17).

_____

_____

_____

God knew the good in me; even though myself and others did not see (Jer. 1:5).

_____

_____

_____

He knew I would be doing what I am doing today! When only God could hear, he was faithful to listen (Isa. 65:24).

_____

_____

_____

When my family was told the devastating news that I may never walk again, God said I would. He uncrippled my body. The Great Physician minded my arm straight again. God returned my feet to a walkable position. The Almighty God repositioned my face so that it regained structure with my voice strained and my speech slurred gone! Sometimes, I speak with a stutter, but I give all the honor, glory, and praise to The Great Physician for my current health.

My God—the God of Abraham, Isaac, and Jacob (Matt. 22:32),

_____

_____

_____

the Creator of the universe in his backyard (Isa. 66:1) saw it fit to give me a wheelchair to glide.

_____

_____

_____

He gave me a walker to take my first step. Then, the Lord said, "I am your crutch. Lean on me, oh daughter, and we will walk." The Great Physician gave me a purple cane and reminded me often that the cane was him (Luke 9:51).

_____

_____

_____

Oh, child of God, when the day came God knew I could labor for him, I left my cane (Ps. 119:133). I proclaimed that I will praise God until my last breath. I'm so happy, cruising with God on this road to recovery. There is no need to look back. There is no room for regret (Luke 9:61–62). It's now only me and the Lord. I choose to allow him to lead my steps (Ps. 139:5). I am still living. I am still recovering. I am still learning. If you are in a struggling battle, take heed; God will take your burden (Ps. 52:32). And just like the good shepherd (Ps. 23), he will carry you too. He is no respecter of persons (Acts 10:34)! What he gives to one, he gives to all.

Today, my health care concerns still exist. I struggle each day with simple tasks. My thoughts are jumbled, and this leaves me with debilitating memory loss. Cognitively, I just can't do the things I used to do, but thank God! He does not call the prequalified; he calls the unqualified to qualify (1 Cor. 1:27).

_____

_____

_____

I continually search in his Word, and now, I'm asked to teach and share the glory God has given me. I find the Word has a unique way of providing what we need each day (Eph. 4:23).

_____

_____

_____

My prayer is that this book will inspire others to use it. My desire is that the lessons reveal answers for the sick, the lame, the blind, the outcast and for each of my brothers and sisters in Christ to gain renewed strength.

I gain strength and find hope in each verse I read (Jer. 29:11).

_____

_____

_____

I'm grateful to the Lord that he has led me to his natural medicine (Ps. 156:6).

_____

_____

_____

I'm encouraged with new faith, as I see others using their Bibles and their essential oils, to improve their lives and the lives of their families! It is an indescribable honor for God to use me, the weakest of you all. The Almighty God gives me my worth, value, and purpose in life (Acts 20:24).

_____

_____

_____

Thank you, for joining me through this journey. For instance, the Holy Bible is my GPS (*God's Plan of Salvation*)! Just like a GPS in a car (Global Positioning Service), Gods instruction book guides me and makes my path straightforward. Therefore, I challenge you to allow your Bible to become your GPS. Let the accounts of the Bible inspire you on your pilgrimage. God's instructions will ensure your lead straight to heaven! I'm praying, this moment, for each of you that pick up this book (Gal. 6:2).

_____

_____

_____

Please God, let their learning challenge my brothers and sisters to carry the Gospel torch (Mark 16:14).

_____

_____

_____

Fill them with your spirit, and give them an opportunity to labor for you.

What are Essential Oils?

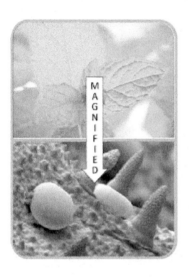

Plant compounds

- Taken from the root, stems, bark, and leaves

- The oils protect the plant from environmental threats

- Our bodies are made of similar building blocks as plants, so when we use oils, they go to work in our bodies in the same way that they would for the plant!

This book does not focus on scientific facts; however, science, theology, and chemistry play a vital role in the success of this book. Average people do not have to understand the chemical compounds with each essential oil to retrieve its benefits. I simply have faith in the Bible and believe God created the essential oils to provide assistance in finding good health. In fact, the Bible is the true Word of God (John 3:3).

With the use of the Saviors' natural medicine, I have witnessed its benefits. I have witnessed the improvement in my family's health, in the health of many of my community members, and in my own body! You see, after my mini-strokes, I had to relearn everything. I have had to learn to totally rely on the Blessed Jesus for everything (Prov. 3:5).

_____

_____

_____

So don't think for a second that I will take the credit for this book.

I use essential oils daily. In the morning, I start with an all-plant-based multivitamins. I blend the following for my digestive issues: ginger, peppermint, tarragon, fennel, caraway, coriander, and anise essential oils. I also use essential oils to clean my home. The essential oils used as cleaning agents are actually better for the health of my family because it leaves out the toxins. The essential oils are the Lord's natural medicine and cleaning agents. Since it is found in our environment it cannot have a patent because we know its origin, and no one person can claim they made the vegetation of the world. The essential oils came by God (Gen. 1). The Messiah (Dan. 9:25)

_____

_____

_____

created the garden (which contained everything man would need in order to survive) before Adam and Eve (Gen. 1:27 and Gen. 2:22).

_____

_____

_____

To have a patent, one must have an original work, and since plants exist naturally, no man can claim their essence. Without getting too technical, the essential oils come from extracting (oils) the essence of plants, resins, and gums in God's backyard (Isa. 66:1).

_____

_____

_____

For example, in 2 Kings 20:7,

_____

_____

_____

God instructed King Hezekiah to harvest fig leaves from God's fig tree. So the king sent a servant to pluck the leaves. The servant knew how to draw out the (oil) essence from the leaves. Ancient people would have crushed the leaves in between two rocks, which would have released the precious oil. Most likely, the servant would have placed the leaves and oils directly on Kings Hezekiah's boils. King Hezekiah was healed of his boils because he obeyed the Redeemer. Today, the favorite method of many is to collect the fig leaves from the Creator's backyard (found where figs grow naturally), boil a pot of water, place the fig leaves in a mason jar, and cook the mason jar full of leaves in the boiling water. Today, one may purchase fig trees from different Internet sites and tree nurseries. Or one may travel to Italy, Turkey, Algeria, Greece, Portugal, or Spain. I have found purchasing oils from my wellness advocate ensures that I'm receiving therapeutic grade oils without all the hassle (www.findhealingingodsbackyard.com).

What Are Therapeutic Grade Oils?

We can all agree that each person has an innermost part (Gen. 2:7).

_____

_____

_____

Most people would agree that their innermost part is the soul. The soul is a portion of our body no man can reach (John 14:6).

_____

_____

_____

So, just like human beings, plants have innermost parts too. The Bible does not say plants have a soul, but we can agree that plants have an essence. Just as humans need blood to thrive (Lev. 17:11),

_____

_____

_____

plants have terpenoids. When you obtain the oils from the leaf's center, you have extracted what is known as the precious oils (Prov. 21:20).

_____

_____

_____

The oil becomes therapeutic grade when the plant is grown in the part of Gods' backyard, where he placed it (Isa. 40:12)

_____

_____

_____

because that is the environment that provides the correct climate and resources for the plant to grow best. Finally, scientists over in France have what they call an ISO certification (ISO standards). ISO chemists seem to have the most reliable chemical constituent indicators. Those standards determine whether an essential oil is therapeutic grade or not.

Examples of Terpenoids:

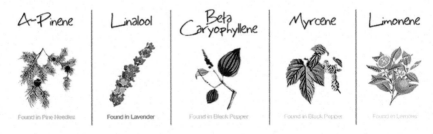

A-Pinene	Linalool	Beta Caryophyllene	Myrcene	Limonene
Found in Pine Needles	Found in Lavender	Found in Black Pepper	Found in Black Pepper	Found in Lemons

The people of scriptural times lived from Italy to Iran and from Greece to Egypt, but a multitude of biblical events occurred in Israel and Palestine. Several botanists allocate the land into five geographic territories. The Israelites lived with sand dunes, coastal plains, fertile soils between the Mediterranean Sea, and hilly plateaus of the east. The people, animals, and plant life had hot, dry summers and extreme winters. Over the years, the landscape changed because much like our culture, the once-fertile land became barren (Isa. 41:18).

God's people cleared the land for timber to fuel fires. The shepherds burned the woodlands to create pastures for domestic animals (Exod. 3:1–3).

Of course, just like today, we have erosion and wastelands (Isa. 5:6) because of wars. Where the essential oil matures naturally is the best way to describe its purity or therapeutic grade oil.

For example, the lilies of the valleys (Song of Sol. 2:1)

---

had extra fragrance for perfume when harvested from coastal areas, rather than gathering the lilies that spring up along the Mediterranean coastline after a long hot dry summer. According to ancient texts, this land would have provided aloes, cumin, spearmint, basil, anise, marjoram, parsley, garlic, dill, chamomile, and many other herbs. Historians believe the inhabitants of the land used the entire root, stem, and leaves. Today, when we distill plants we use machinery to press and grind.

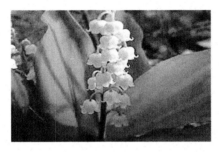

Template of what the lily of the valley may resembled.

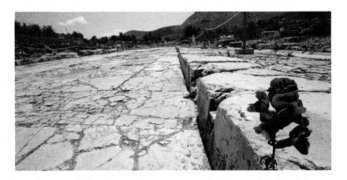

Vegetation in Jerusalem.

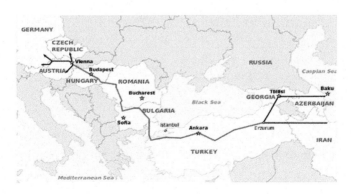

Territory Map

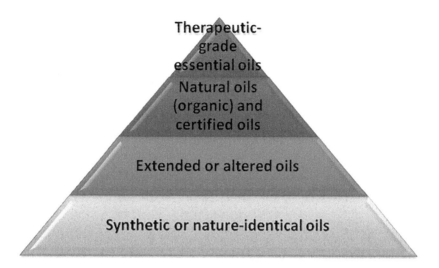

The crucial action in generating a therapeutic grade essential oil is to reserve numerous amounts of delicate aromatic compounds within the oil. Countless numbers of these elements are very fragile and are slaughtered by hot temperature and extraordinary pressure. The process of distillation often is the determining factor in the value of the oil. Essential oil distilling is hard work and somewhat a form of art. The owner of the distillery must understand heat and pressure. If the pressure is too elevated or the temperature is too extreme, it may change the molecular structure and affect the products fragrance; thus, altering the products' chemical constituents.

What Is Aromatherapy?

God the Creator is a remarkable scientist who understand the scientific process of everything that exists in world (Rev. 22:13).

_____

_____

_____

Aromatherapists, botanists, holistic doctors, and reflexologist can be described as the professionals who handle essential oils and therapy. This group of scientists utilize the plant's aroma-producing fragments (essential oils) to treat many different illnesses and diseases. Most Christians recognize (2 Tim. 3:1)

_____

_____

_____

that society requires aromatherapists and other art forms to explain and model techniques that would lead to better health. Currently, herbalism medicine routinely studies God's backyard to determine what plant can be harvested. Botanists harvest the core of flowers, leaves, stalks, gums, resins, rinds, roots, etc. Scientists creatively combine these different substances to create God's medicine. Ezekiel 47:12 states,

_____

"By the river upon the bank thereof, on this side and on that side, shall grow all trees for meat, whose leaf shall not fade, neither shall the fruit thereof be consumed: it shall bring forth new fruit according to his months, because their waters they issued out of the sanctuary: and the fruit thereof shall be for meat, and the leaf thereof for medicine." Subsequently, when Christians combine essential oils with prayer, miracles transpire (James 5:14).

Only chemists, holistic doctors, aromatherapist, and skilled perfumers should combine essential oils. No one else should blend his or her own concoctions. The best way to educate yourself on the implementation of essential oils is to complete this study, attend a class or two offered by a wellness advocate, visit doctors, examine current research, and watch educational videos. According to the Bible (Mark 16:13),

the disciples drove out many demons, anointed many sick people with oil and healed them. Aromatherapists are experts at using the essential oils as medicine (1 John 2:1).

Aromatherapists and holistic doctors are proficient. These professionals school the general population on how to implement essential oils in our daily lives. For example, through education, society can learn how to use essential oils topically, internally, and by diffusion.

According to aromatherapists, when essential oils are diffused, their molecules are absorbed in our air passages, creating healing properties for the body. Another clever method to utilize essential oils is by pouring them into bath water. According to many scriptures of the Bible, God's children used the method of pouring oils onto their bodies. This action of pouring on the oils is similar to the way we pour oils in the bathtub because in the ancient days, there was no running water. I can picture Anna (Luke 2:37),

_____

_____

_____

Jael (Judg. 4),

_____

_____

Abigail (1 Sam. 25), Lois, and Eunice (2 Tim. 1:5)

_____

_____

pouring in oils of rose and hyssop in their baths. King Herod had several public pools of water, and they've been discovered by archaeologists. His bathing area included dressing rooms and separate courts for male and female. He even had some built-in baths his living quarters. He modeled his courts after the Romans. However, in most scriptures, the pouring on of oil was done for the purpose of anointing.

According to Exodus 29:7,

_____

_____

_____

take the anointing oil, and anoint him by pouring it on his head. Practitioners of aromatherapy believe that fragrances in the oils stimulate nerves in the nose. The nerves send impulses to the part of the brain that controls memory and emotion. Christians agree, according to the Bilbe, that people are healed by the work of the Author and Perfecter of our faith (Heb. 12:2).

_____

_____

_____

Whichever way you believe, I'm glad both ideas merge into one, and I have witnessed the benefits of consuming essential oils.

The Great Creator made us distinctively. Therefore, God had to produce several different species of plants. Gods' people extracted essential oils, and a blessing from the Father healed multiple sicknesses. Jeremiah 27:5 states,

_____

_____

_____

"Before I formed thee in the belly I knew thee; and before thou camest forth out of the womb I sanctified thee, and I ordained thee a prophet unto the nations." Deliverance from a sickness depends on many differentiations. The formation of each individual person is different; therefore, the results are common but continually vary between people. The variations depended on the type of essential oil consumed and the symptoms of the patient. The result on the body may have be calming or stimulating. I've witnessed one oil blend working for one person but not as well on the second person. Thus, this can be explained in God's Word because he made us all different for all different reasons. Romans 12:6 says we have different gifts according to the grace given to each of us. If your gift is prophesying, then prophesy in accordance with your faith. In addition, a couple of theories in science indicate that the oils react with the body's hormones and enzymes. Scientists educate that hormones and enzymes can change blood pressures, pulses, and moods. In another scientific theory, holistic physicians suggest that the fragrance from several oils may stimulate the body to produce pain-fighting substances. It's because of those theories I began using essential oils. I've witnessed their effectiveness. I quickly realized something was missing. God led me to the scriptures. I awoke every morning connecting his Word and fell asleep in utterance with Jesus. I recommend using essential oils not because scientists promote them, but because God ordained their use.

Eight AROMATHERAPY Scents

ROSEMARY

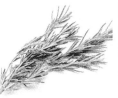

Thought to stimulate the brain and mental performance.

PEPPERMINT

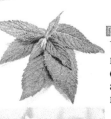

Used to relieve mental fatigue, enhance alertness, and enhance memory.

LEMON

The uplifting aroma of lemon has been known to enhance mental clarity and reduce stress and depression.

EUCALYPTUS

Most commonly used to open the sinuses and bronchial passages. Also used to relieve headaches and mental fatigue.

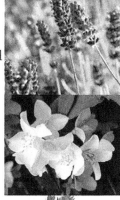

LAVENDER

One of the most widely used oils, lavender is uplifitng and relaxing.

JASMINE

Used to fight stress and anxiety.

THYME

May help improve memory and concentration. Also known to relax the nervous system.

SANDALWOOD

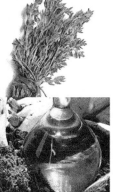

Used to calm the nerves and induce relaxation.

Can Essential Oils Provide Relief
for Depression and Anxiety?

Since my life has been inverted with sickness, I recommend God's medicine to anyone who will hear his Word. For example, I have suffered from depression for many years. I've been prescribed many different medications, but recently, I've seen an improvement with the use of emotional blends of oils. For example, essential oils like peppermint, lemon, orange, sandalwood, grapefruit, tangerine, and lavender have kept my mood elevated. The smell of sandalwood, when inhaled, provides immediate relief of my depression symptoms. Now, when I hear the word sandalwood, I smile. I don't use all these oils at one time, but I defuse them, drink some of them in water, massage them along my temples, and soak with them in my bathtub. Exhausting the essential oils in the manner has influenced my mental well-being for the better. The author or anyone connected to this book does not suggest that you stop taking your prescriptions and seek medical treat for any suicidal tendencies (Exod. 20:13).

_____

_____

_____

Search the scriptures, and you'll locate several people suffering from depression. For example, Naomi in the book of Ruth was depressed because she recognized her separation of all she ever appreciated. Have you ever moved? I've never moved out of my home state of West Virginia. But whether you move out of town or across town, it's all stressful. Naomi's move was more than stressful; her move was permanent! I just don't know if I could leave all that I've ever owned behind. Another example of a depressed person in biblical days was Hannah (1 Sam. 1; 2:1, 21).

_____

_____

_____

Hannah was an amazing mother. She was a true character of faith and was the perfect example of patience. Her life circumstances were truly depressing, but then, God came and gave her victory. God provided Hannah with a boy name Samuel. A barren woman in Hannah's day was tragic because a large family was understood to truly be blessed of God. The male child was significant because men were considered the higher being, and family histories were traced through the male. Hannah kept her promise to God. After raising him from birth, when he was of age, she gave God her son. Samuel went down in biblical history as a faithful servant recorded in Hebrews 11:32.

_____

_____

_____

Many more people of the Bible era suffered with depression symptoms. A few to mention were King Solomon, Moses, John the Baptist, Saul who became Paul, Jeremiah, and, of course, Job. Mental health providers will inform you that depression can affect everyone, and our Bible confirms this statement. People from all walks of life can suffer with depression. Depression can affect the fruitful, the deprived, the adolescent, the elderly, the gentleman, and the female. We find several examples in scripture today. King Solomon was affluent among his people, and some say he had everything. But depression overtook him. Deprived people like Ruth and Naomi saw their portion of death and sorrow. Adolescent men of the Bible like David and Job were for sure aggrieved with depression. Even mother Mary was heartbroken and miserable at the sight of her Son, being beaten and put to death. Finally, Hannah was barren, and Jeremiah was known as the weeping prophet.

The good news is that essential oils contain healing properties to lift and stabilize our moods. I wonder what Jesus's family blended together to help Mary. I wonder if Hannah kept lilies, roses, and lilacs on her table. I wonder when Naomi anointed herself for Boaz if she was influenced emotionally. I wonder if David the shepherd found wild flowers to smell. I bet weeping prophet Jeremiah kept a depression essential oil blend in his dwelling place. The scriptures communicate that we must be prepared and have essential oils on hand. We know that God's people knew the verse form Proverbs well. Proverbs 21:20 says, "There is treasure to be desired and oil in the dwelling of the wise; but a foolish man spendeth it up." Everyone desires to be considered intelligent. Everyone bestows advice and nobody hungers to be considered a fool. So remember the purpose of this scripture. The action of storing oils in your home is a wise decision. Possibly, warehousing essential oils is a wise decision, because of all the health benefits! Since, I've started teaching lessons (that God allows) more and more people (saved and unsaved) contact me for essential oils. So I definitely, want to be prepared to comfort the sick. Be advised that our God is in control. God distributes exactly what we require and dispatches those who possess a willing heart (Matt. 6:24).

Give heed to his word and keep investigating (2 Tim. 2:15).

_____

_____

_____

Why Is Essential Oil Valuable?

Modern medicine would like to have people believe that there is no value in alternative medicine, but in the Bible, we discovery different news. Examining the scriptures, we realize essential oils are valuable because we find God's original medicine being used daily. From creation in Genesis 1:29–30, we read that Creator God made plants for our nourishment and medical needs.

_____

_____

_____

Based on these scriptures alone, we should be convinced that essential oils are valuable, and we should use them in our daily routines. In the book of James, he explains that we should pray, and we should have the elders of the church pray with us. James tells us to use our prayer line for the healing of our bodies, souls, and minds. Christians would be obeying God's Word if we would all learn to trust him.

The people of biblical times used essential oils daily. Presently, an abundance of people are understanding the healthcare benefits. In biblical days, essential oils provided nutrition and made food taste better. The essential oils were used as incense in the home, in businesses, for hospitality, and in the synagogue. In worship, the odor of the incenses provided a way for the Jews to identify God. The pouring on of the essential oils notified God's people of his chosen leader. Moreover, the essential oils were very expensive and precious to the people. Research the scriptures of Song of Solomon 4:10 and John 12:3, because these two verses explain why the essential oils were expensive and precious.

_____

_____

_____

Song of Solomon New Living Translation: "Your love delights me, my treasure, my bride. Your love is better than wine, your perfume more fragrant than spices." According to this scripture, in this chapter, Jesus Christ explains our value to him. The church who believes in him is valuable because the church depends on him; they continue to be influenced by his grace, and this makes us more acceptable to him (Ps. 91:14).

_____

_____

_____

John 12:3 says,

_____

_____

_____

"Then Mary took a twelve-ounce jar of expensive perfume made from essence of nard, and she anointed Jesus' feet with it, wiping his feet with her hair. The house was filled with the fragrance." Consequently, the chapter is a continuation of the previous chapter in dishonoring Jesus. The dishonor given to Lord Jesus was when the scribes and Pharisees proclaimed Jesus to be a traitor. However, in verse 3 of the chapter, we find Mary awarding Jesus with her admiration. The sinner illustrated her reverence for him by anointing his feet at dinner in Bethany. Here is a tidbit for thought: I will not call anyone reverend because no one but Jesus deserves the tile (1Sam. 2:2, Rom. 3:23, Gal. 6:3).

_____

_____

_____

Finally, the actions of Mary contradicted the thoughts of the Pharisees and Scribes. We understand, through this account, that the essential oil of myrrh and her actions gave honor to our Redeemer. We should heap honor and humiliation on the head of the Lord Jesus.

Furthermore, the oils of cedarwood, frankincense, and myrrh were also valuable to the Jews because these oils were combined and spent in burial proceedings. In addition, Numbers 9:11 says,

_____

_____

_____

"On the fourteenth day of the second month at even they shall keep it, and eat it with unleavened bread and bitter herbs." Exodus 12:8 also says,

_____

_____

_____

"And they shall eat the flesh in that night, roast with fire, and unleavened bread; and with bitter herbs they shall eat it." The bitter herbs could have been chamomile, hyssop, galbanum, or wormwood because these herbs would have been harvested in their environment.

These oils had value to God's people because the plants added flavor to their food and symbolized a different mystical meaning.

The Almighty, instructed his people to use his blend to anoint God's chosen shepherds. Read 1 Samuel 10:1,

_____

_____

_____

Numbers 27:18,

_____

_____

_____

Leviticus 21:10,

_____

_____

_____

1 Kings 1:39

_____

_____

_____

Through investigation, acknowledgement will conclude essential oils were used in biblical anointings. In addition, Hebrews were to anoint many other things. In the book of Samuel, the tenth chapter and eighteenth verse, we see Samuel anoints Saul. According to biblegateway.com, "Then Samuel took a flask of olive oil and poured it over Saul's head. He kissed Saul and said, 'I am doing this because the LORD HAS APPOINTED YOU TO BE THE RULER OVER ISRAEL, HIS SPECIAL POSSESSION.'" VISUALIZE, SAMUEL and Saul walking together over hills, in grazing fields, passing a shepherd or two, and over several fields before arriving at Ramah. I can see the vineyards of botanicals and the fields of grazing land. Arriving at the congregation of the Jews, I can see them receiving a warm welcome and the anointing Saul. Definitely, on this day, the essential oils had sufficient value for God and his people.

In 1 Kings 1:39, it states, "Then Zadok the priest took a horn of oil from the tabernacle and anointed Solomon. And they blew the horn, and all the people said, 'Long live King Solomon!'" Since he was a younger son, he was made king by divine appointment. I suspect his title was somewhat contested! For this reason, the pouring on the oil of gladness symbolized the qualification of Christ. He was the anointed one—meaning, the Spirit was poured on Solomon. King Solomon was in fact the next chosen leader of God's people. This thrills my heart, and I hope you understand the upmost value of oil. Grab your Bible, and turn to Hebrews 1:9 and Psalm 89:20.

_____

_____

_____

All Christians, being *heirs of the kingdom* do from him (Christ) *receive the anointing* (1 John 2:27).

_____

_____

_____

Sisters, we are God's chosen ones! Definitely, after reviewing the above verses, we find another meaning. All the military were ordered to give the public notice of the new King. The people were to express their joy publicly. They announced this with a trumpet as they did on several accounts in the Bible. Do you remember confessing Jesus when you were saved (Rom. 10:9)? Finally, at the end of the verse, it states "*Let king Solomon live!*"—announcing their prayer for him to prosper, thus, establishing God's kingdom under his rule. This is absolutely similar to the jubilee we have in church services when the spirit is felt or someone accepts Jesus. Ultimately, this gives us an inside view to why we place the new pastor's name on the marquee. Can you recall a time your church searched for a pastor, and the time of celebration that came when the anointed one arrived? I can fathom this huge idea in my mind's eye. How awesome!

How Were God's People
Saturated in Essential Oils?

According to Genesis 50 and Exodus 2, in the land of Egypt, God's people were held as prisoners, as slaves (Exod. 5:1).

_____

_____

_____

Egyptians are considered distinguished experts for embalming their dead. Enslaved Israelites may possibly be instructed on the process of mummification. We all understand there is life, and there is death. The enemy of death occurs daily. Israelites were submerged in Egyptian culture. In fact, enslaved Israelites were probably in charge of burying the Egyptians and Israelites.

John 19:40 states, "Taking Jesus' body, the two of them wrapped it, with the spices, in strips of linen."

_____

_____

_____

So we see here the process of mummification was still a customs of the Jews. The plan of the Israelites was to take the body of Jesus, use oil and spices, and wrap him in linen cloths. We also know that Mary and Martha did this for Lazarus because in John 11:44 states,

---

"The dead man [Lazarus] came out, his hands and feet were wrapped with strips of linen, and a cloth around his face. Jesus said to them, 'Take off the grave clothes and let him go.'"

Another Jewish custom during biblical days was feet washing. The Israelites harvested fragrant oils to wash the feet of their guest. When a friend or family member had traveled from a far distance, there feet were washed upon arrival. In the biblical era, they usually walked barefoot or wore sandals. Because of the bad terrain, the guest often arrived with cuts and bruises on their feet. Running water was not available; therefore, a large pottery bowl of essential oils and water were offered to the exhausted guest. For example, the following essential oils have assisted several people: sandalwood, fennel, lavender, geranium, rosewood, rosemary, myrtle, and cedarwood; these would have been the most obtainable oils. The people of ancient times were excellent aromatherapists. Since hygiene and germs were an issue, they would have chosen a blend with aloes and eucalypts that were both fragrant and soothing to the feet.

According to Genesis 24:32, feet washing was a true custom. In fact, the action of feet washing was a norm among the Jews. In Genesis 24:32, a man came to the house and unharnessed the camels, and gave straw and fodder to the camels, and there was *water to wash his feet* and the feet of the men who were with him. According to The Amplified Bible, the man's name was Laban. According the genealogy in Genesis, Laban was the brother in law of Isaac and the uncle of Jacob. In addition, when mother Mary traveled to Elizabeth's home,

I wonder if her feet were washed by Elizabeth. What a pleasure would that have been! According to the philosophy of a reflexologist, your entire body can be reached through your feet. I wonder if Elizabeth placed pebbles in the bottom of the bowl to relax her tired soul. I assume aloes were provided after the foot spa because an experienced reflexologists massages lotion on the feet after drying.

Long ago, societies were drawn to essential oils. History has proven the healing powers for earth's inhabitants. Today, societies are relearning how effective essential oils are for improving emotions and for improving focus. Moses's nation used essential oils in their worship of God too. According to the Bible, the holy anointing oil identified God's people. For example, in Exodus 30:22–25,

_____

_____

_____

The Israelites were instructed to burn holy incense in the temple. When the Israelites entered to the synagogue, the aroma from God's extraordinary blend produced a fragrant aroma. The perfumed aroma signaled God was in the midst of the temple. The odor occupied the entire tabernacle. As the children of God exited the meeting tent, the distinct aroma attached to their clothing and was carried along all day. Finally, as the Jews congregated to the city court, they effortlessly recognized one another. I've heard it said, "I know you are a Jew because you smell like one." All of the enemies of the Jews could also recognize them.

John 15:8 states,

_____

_____

_____

In our society, people are recognized as Christians by the harvest they bring. John 15:8 (NIV) states, "This is to my Father's glory that you bear much fruit, showing yourselves to be my disciples." Christians are also identified according to their conversation and possessions. For example, Christians place images of Christ on their automobiles and on personal items they wear. For instance, masses of people have licenses plates with the name of Jesus. Some automobiles have auto decals of Christian symbols. Some of the Christian icons are fish, crosses, praying hands, or the Christian flags. Finally, Christians also wear cross jewelry and meet at the church; however, I've never heard you smell like a Christian.

Let's examine why people associate a fish with Christ. In ancient days, when two Jews meet, one would draw half of a fish on the ground with his or her feet. Then, they would wait to see if the other person would draw the other half of the fish. If the other person did not draw the fish, the Jew did not openly talk to them about Christ. The picture is known as an Ichthys. The acronym IXEYO, which comes from a Greek term, means "Jesus Christ God's Son is Savior." This idea steams from the ancient scriptures where fish are mentioned. In the Holy Bible, the word fish is referenced many times. To prove this notion, please read the following scriptures:

Matthew 4:19,

_____

_____

_____

Mark 6,

_____

_____

_____

Luke 9,

_____

_____

_____

John 6,

_____

_____

_____

What about Just Prayer Alone?

Essential oil in the Word of God becomes powerful when we combine essential oils with prayer. Prayers and oils generate fabulous reactions. In Leviticus 8:10,

_____

_____

_____

Moses used the anointing oil to sanctify and purify. He poured the oil on the altar seven times. God also instructed the king or ruler to anoint the head of God's next chosen leader. Today, as a child of God, in accordance to the Bible, we are able to use the anointing oil as a symbol of Christ's blood. The action of praying and anointing ourselves with oil imitates the anointing of Christ on our body. In prayer, asking God for an anointing is comparable to calling on the Holy Spirit for guidance.

The scriptures report God's anointed people practiced this custom and God bequeathed miracles. In the book of Ruth chapter 1, Ruth told Naomi to wash herself, put the anointing oil on and go and lay at Boaz's feet. Then, Boaz took her to become his wife. Many scholars believe this to be an act of obedience. The anointing Naomi received was not only smelling great, but she was anointed with the blessing of God. A foreigner became welcome in marriage to a noble heart that followed God. She was poor, not knowing day to day what was going to happen, to becoming wealthy and living in an environment of love and kindness. Overall, Ruth and Naomi had faith in God and he blessed them above measure. Below are two modern ways we can use prayer and anointing oil.

The first way to use essential oils is to wash your home with oils and wash your body with the oil.

1 John 4:1 states,

_____

_____

_____

Second, today, for example, each morning, after showering, I place essential oils on my feet, right up to my knees; as I massage on the oil (anointing myself), I pray for the Lord's protection. Sometimes, I deploy the same oil recipe because the aroma is pleasing, but on other occasions, I choose an oil formula to treat an obstruction. Choose oils to help your skin condition. For example, I might combine melaleuca and lavender if I have a rash. For eczema, you can try lavender, patchouli, and bergamot. Add clove and clary sage to both the water and moisturizer to increase memory. As you pray, request to be drenched in the Holy Spirit. So you can withstand in the wicked ways of the world. The world is polluted with defilements contrary to the Word. As you voyage on the roads of life, corruption will stick to the souls of your feet. Through our feet, the entire body could be defiled, and we could pass the tarnishing onto unaware contacts. So pray daily for God's protection and guidance. In addition, please take heed of God's Word and finish this walk with Bible clearly. An essential oil for clarity is rosemary. Rosemary has a fabulous aroma when defused in the air. Rosemary can be applied to the temples and neck.

Prayers for Spiritual Healing

The Good Book explains in Matthew chapter 6 the process and necessity of prayer. Jesus directly instructs us to pray in a certain manner. Matthew 6:9–13 consummates a standard in the method we must pray. First, we ought to know who our Father is and where he lives. We must show admiration for him. Second, we should tell him that we worship him with a thankful heart. Third, we should confess our sin. Fourth, we should deliver our petitions. Finally, we should trust him to care for us and thank him for answering our prayer.

When we pray, God occasionally will not listen. For example, John 9:31 says, "Now we know that God heareth not sinners: but if any man be a worshipper of God, and doeth his will, him he heareth." This part of scripture is sour to the belly, but 2 Corinthians 6:2 (KJV) states, "For he saith, I have heard thee in a time accepted, and in the day of salvation have I succoured thee: behold, now is the accepted time; behold, now is the day of salvation." The present is the day to be saved. God is everywhere, so we do not have to be at an altar to be saved. God saves people on vacation, at home, in cars, outside, in the hospital, and everywhere. Romans 10:9 states, "If you declare with your mouth, 'Jesus is Lord,' and believe in your heart that God raised him from the dead, you will be saved." Then, Isiah 65:24 states, "And it shall come to pass, that before they call, I will answer; and while they are yet speaking, I will hear." This is the best prayer because God cleans you inside and out. Christ provides healing for the body, soul, and mind (2 Cor. 5:17).

_____

_____

_____

In the Word, we find an example in Matthew. It's here we find a story of the faith with the Canaanite woman. Matthew 15:26–28 states, "But Jesus replied, 'It is not right to take the children's bread and toss it to the dogs (v. 26).' 'Yes, Lord,' she said, 'even the dogs eat the crumbs that fall from their master's table (v. 27).' 'O woman,' Jesus answered, 'your faith is great! Let it be done for you as you desire.' And her daughter was healed from that very hour (v. 28)." The mother requesting Jesus to heal her daughter had to get right (repent) before Jesus could heal her daughter. My mother, Becky, claims this verse because all those nights in the hospital, not knowing if I'm coming back from my strokes or not, she spoke to God. But this verse entered her mind. Thank God, he saved her and healed me. I'm sure the women in the verse also felt the same way. If my mother and I only recognized God's medicine at that time. I now understand I would have received quicker relief of my symptoms, and my mother may not have felt so helpless because she would have been the applying them to my skin (anointing) and praying.

Prayer Essentials

_____

_____

_____

Prayer Essentials

A preacher once commented to me that we are only as strong as our prayer life. God actually speaks to us through his Word. His word is recorded in a book called the Bible. So we have the book. Does that mean God wants to speak to us? Yes, but oftentimes, we ignore him. We do not read his conversation. When we pray we talk to God. A personal relationship can't grow with anyone if we can talk to them. So if there is no communication, there can't be a relation with Christ.

A Christian's prayer doesn't have to be complex. During this study, you will be asked to write prayers to our Savior, so below are several selected tips. You can add more tips as you go through this study. If you're seeking God in prayer, I suggest the following ideas:

- *Be aware.* Ask yourself what are you needing and who are you praying for. Always know who you are praying to.
- *Be honest.* Be honest and open with God. He only hears your heart anyway.
- *Repent if you need to.* Confess your sin! Ask for forgiveness and help!
- *Don't rush.* When you pray when you're alone, picture Jesus sitting across from you.
- *Be thankful.* Honor God with praise. Be at peace for the prayer has been answered. Below is a graphic organizer to show how the above tips can be put to work in God's Word.

	Reviewing the Lord's Prayer	
God -------------	Our Father which art in heaven, Hallowed be thy name. Thy kingdom come, Thy will be done in earth, as it is in heaven.	---------- Worship--------- ---------Allegiance--------- ----------Petition ----------
Jesus ------------	Give us this day our daily bread. And forgive us our debts, as we forgive our debtors. And lead us	
Holy Ghost -------	not into temptation, but deliver us from evil: For thine is the kingdom, and the power, and the glory, forever. Amen.	--------Confession-------- --------Deliverance-------

Anointing Is a Bible Term

To anoint, according to Oxford Dictionaries (Oxford University Press, translation by Bing Translator) is a verb that means *to smear or rub with oil*, typically as part of a religious ceremony:

> For methods of hospitably, sanitization, and fragrances.
> To bring physical healing of plagues, ailments, and disease.
> "High priests were anointed with oil."
> "He was anointed as the organizational candidate of the party."
> Pouring essential oils over the heads of people to show reverence and contentment.
> Dipping or pouring essential oils on tangible items to set them apart as God's instruments.
> "Bodies were anointed after death for burial."
> In preparation of a bride in marriage.
> To bring legal change through new agreements.
> "The disciples and Jesus casted out devils."
> Metaphorically, to represent the change in an unclean heart to purified heart.

Origin

Middle English: from Old French *enoint* "anointed," past participle of *enoindre*, from Latin *inungere*, from *in* (upon) + *ungere* (anoint, smear with oil).

Anointing oil is referred as an unguent in scientific lingo. Biblical times anointing oil was often referred to just as an ointment. In fact, the word anoint appears more than 156 times. In ancient days, the anointing oil was prepared from oil alone and often with the addition of flowers, fragrant herbs, gums, resins, seeds, spices, and other botanicals. For this reason, flower gardens were popular. For instance, for a reference, search the scriptures for King Solomon's gardens. Some formulas were very simple and consisted of one active ingredient and olive oil; however, some essential oil formulas were complex mixtures of ingredients. These unguent or ointments had distinct aromatic odors: earthy, spicy, herbal, medicinal, balsamic, or sweet aromas. The term *anointing oil* did not always describe a sweet memorizing fragrance. Anointing oils were used for different reasons and were not always like the perfumes we buy at the store today.

We perceive in Matthew 26:7

and John 12:3–8

that the oils are known as precious ointment. The precious ointment existed as the costliest medicine to the ancient people. The Precious oils that transpired were myrrh, frankincense, and spikenard. Moreover, in Mark 6:13, the ointment was used to drive away demons.

In John 9:11, the scripture used mud of the ancient world to cure blindness.

The power of prayer definitely granted the healing. I can't find anyone that has rubbed mud on their eyes and now they can see. Jesus could have healed him minus the mud, but the Jews (and us today) always needed a sign.

The truth is that the Christians and the world has lost the meaning of anoint with oil. In modern times, most ministers anoint the sick, in accordance to James, with one or two drops of oil. The oils, on average, are a fatty oil, like vegetable or olive, purchased from a local grocery store. Most of the time, churches use olive because the word olive appears more in the New Testament. I've even witnessed churches using mineral oil. Mineral oil contains petroleum, and it could be potentially harmful. It encourages me to understand all good things come down from above (James 1:17).

In addition, according to the Bible, priests were the only ones to make medicine for leprosy. Frankincense was used in the essential oil blend for leprosy because it would have given the recipient a soothing feel. In the Bible, we see lots of leprosy victims pursuing a cure. For example, recorded in Luke 17:12, 13,

_____

_____

_____

Jesus heals the ten and sends them back to the priests because it was the law at that time that no one could use God's special formula that contained frankincense for personal use.

In history books, Jews did not just apply a couple of drops to someone's forehead. The biblical practice was to pour the oil on the head. The head was massaged. Prayers for the person was brought by the children of God in the form of petitions. The oil actually ran down the face and beard and onto the clothing. In those days, hygiene was lacking, and the oil would have provided a pleasant odor and a shield from germs.

The most common biblical act modern Christians associate with the word anoint is in the action of anointing. Many churches only refer to the term anoint in one scripture. This scripture comes from the book of James. James instructs the sick to call on the elders of the church, be anointed with oil, and ask God for the healing. However, it's interesting that James did not say do this in the temple. But the temple has become the place our society has determined to be where healings occur. I challenge you, as you complete the lessons in this manual, that you also use God's blend to anoint right in your class. The power is not in just dropping a couple drops of oil onto someone's forehead as stated above. Moreover, this action has a greater meaning in symbolism. God's medicine is not in just one oil or in one application. God's medicine came in various forms because there are several different types of essential oils and several different illnesses to treat. For example, if I were being anointed for a backache it would make more sense to massage five drops of peppermint, rosemary, and basil or cassia on the sore area, then just to drop a couple drop of plain olive oil onto my forehead. The combining of peppermint, rosemary, and basil is God's medicine, and when blended, it produces a pain reliever. Prayer is needed to magnify God's medicine. The following is an example prayer that will help you understand what anointing is and how to apply the concept to your own life.

Pour on your essential oil, blend, and pray:

Sample One (Spiritual)

In the name of Jesus, I proclaim that this no longer is just an essential oil. The essential oil blend represents the blood Jesus Christ shed on Calvary for me. I commit this essential oil blend to you, Lord. I place your power and authority over my life. I ask, Lord, that you anoint me with your power and with the Holy Spirit.

Amen.

Sample Two (Physical)

In the name of Jesus, I proclaim that this essential oil blend is no longer just a mixture of essential oils but the blood of Jesus Christ. Father, I ask that you place your power on whomever or whatever I place this essential oil blend upon. Lord, I ask that you please send your special healing miracles today. Lord, at this moment, give us deliverance and cleansing by your Holy Ghost. We claim all these petitions as being delivered in the name of Jesus.

Amen.

Of course, the Bible suggests anointment of the spirit in Psalm 2:2,

_____

_____

_____

which for us is in the example oil above! We also find more references to anointment of the spirit in Lamentations 4:20,

Ezekiel 28:14,

Habakkuk 3:13,

Zechariah 4:14,

Luke 4:18,

Acts 4:27, and more.

For example, Psalm 23 describes a spiritual annointing. Of course, one of the lessons include a detailed study of the chapter. Psalm 23:5 states,

_____

_____

_____

"Thou preparest a table before me in the presence of mine enemies: thou anointest my head with oil; my cup runneth over." Then what is recorded? Psalm 23:6 states,

_____

_____

_____

"Surely goodness and mercy shall follow me all the days of my life: and I will dwell in the house of the Lord forever." In addition, anointing was also on things and not people. Investigate the following scriptures:

Genesis 35:14,

_____

_____

_____

2 Samuel 1:21,

_____

_____

_____

and Isaiah 21:5 for more references.

_____

_____

_____

God's Own Special Blend

Examine the Holy Scriptures for the holy anointing incense. Begin in
Exodus 30: 34–35 and Exodus 29:2.

_____

_____

_____

In conclusion, the scriptures reveal the pouring on of oil in the following scriptures: Exodus 29:7,

_____

_____

_____

Leviticus 8:10–12,

_____

_____

_____

1 Samuel 10:1,

_____

_____

_____

Leviticus 21:10,

_____

_____

_____

and 2 Kings 9:6.

_____

_____

_____

Israelites used the pouring method by the action of pouring on the oils over the head. The oils poured over the head were rejuvenating. The best picture of this is best understood from the book of Exodus 30:34–35, God instructs Moses to create a special blend: "Also unto thee principal spices, of pure myrrh five hundred shekels, and of sweet cinnamon half so much, even two hundred and fifty shekels, and of sweet calamus two hundred and fifty shekels, And of cassia five hundred shekels, after the shekel of the sanctuary, and of oil olive an hin." This blend made together created the holy anointing oil. Then, later in Exodus, God gives instructions for how to use the anointing oil. I adore that God created the plants essence and that he told us the procedures to improve our relationship with him. God himself proclaimed the essential oils to heal our bodies. I'm especially joyful to comprehend that God created his own holy combination.

At this time in biblical history, the Israelites were motionless in the desert. They were traveling to the Promised Land when the Lord commanded Moses to construct he holy anointing oil and incense. The anointing oil was used for consecrating the high priest and his sons, the altar, the Ark of the Covenant, and the tent meetings. The High Priest at this time would have been Aaron. Finally, in accordance to God's instructions, Aaron offered the fragrant incense formulated in Exodus 30:34–35 on the altar every morning and evening.

The burning of God's blend and the anointing of God's combination didn't end in the desert. The desert was just the beginning. After the temple was built in Jerusalem, incense was offered to God on the golden altar and at the Holy veil. Luke 1:8–10 records that when the priest came into the sanctuary of the Lord, incense was offered as people prayed outside.

_____

_____

_____

We read later detailed accounts of God's chosen leaders being anointed. In Jesus's day, we see Jesus giving healings. On the other hand, early Christians didn't burn incense because of the pagan connotations and the persecution days of the disciples. Christians were also told to burn incense to the Roman emperors and their gods. Later, in the Jewish tradition, ritual cleansing of ancient objects was as anointing for the faithful to symbolize sanctification.

One final thought, the formula had a secret ingredient not known to this author. The cryptic formulas were only created by the best professional perfumers because this one essential oil could have been an herb; it produced smoke that did not fill the room. The smoke made a direct beam straight up, maybe pointing to heaven.

According to the Gospel of Mark 6:13,

_____

_____

_____

Jesus went around, teaching from village to village. He always called the twelve disciples to go with him. In this chapter of the

Bible, Jesus begins to send the twelve out two by two, and he gave them authority over impure spirits. Mark 6:13 says, "They drove out many demons and anointed many sick people with oil and healed them." Mark does not elaborate on the content of the oils used by the disciples. But he did not have to because at time, it was normal for the people to use aromatic ingredients. When an anointing oil was referred to, it was simply stated as oil, but it was understood by the people of that time that the carrier oil was either olive or myrrh. The Jews knew for the vital essences of the aromatics was contained in the anointing. Using a vegetable base oil as a carrier oil allowed the disciples to use their stock of essential oils more cost effectively. Using the blend of oils enabled the disciples to share God's medicine with more people.

What Is a Prayer Cloth?

There are several biblical accounts that are the basis of this modern practice. Christians believe that a prayer cloth assists the recipient in receiving positive answers to prayer. This tradition was instigated with this resulting occurrence. In the book of Matthew, we observe the story of a woman who had suffered severe bleeding for twelve years (Matt. 9:20–22).

_____

_____

_____

She had spent all she had on prescriptions and physicians but still was not heard. She undoubtedly heard about Jesus. She managed to touch the hem of Jesus's cloak, believing this simple contact would heal her. Jesus answered in verse 22, telling her, "Your faith has made you well." Also, in Matthew 14:34–36, the people of Gennesaret had a similar thought.

_____

_____

_____

Absolutely all the sick heard the fame of Jesus and desired to touch only the hem of Jesus's garment. We have the duty to advertise that Jesus's apparel was never tattered. The interpretation found in

Acts 19:11–12 conveys the message of how the handkerchiefs that Paul had merely caressed were carried to the sick, in hopes that people would be healed of diseases and evil spirits.

Paul never termed his handkerchief a "prayer cloth." The New Testament missionaries were extremely hardworking. The preachers were doing a labor of love for Christ. The teachers were underneath pressure to deliver the Gospel to an innumerable number of people. The tradition was that kinsmen would rip a piece of fabric from their Paul's sweatband. Then, the public would tear pieces of cloth. The believers would distribute the miniature piece of fabric to the sick. The unwell individual that accepted the textile was restored according to their faith.

In biblical times, gentiles had no designation for this practice. The first contemporary use of a prayer cloth may have been by the Mormons. When, the practice diminished in Mormonism, it flourished in the Pentecostal church. Today, the tradition may be instituted in the Roman Catholic churches and throughout Christian Churches across the United States. Currently, the prayer cloth is not anointed with sweat from those who pray over it, but rather it's anointed with a fatty oil like vegetable. As more Christians learn how to use original medicine for healing, we can predict more churches will use essential oils with a mood stabilizer. Churches could use vegetable oil but also include citrus or peppermint to boost happy feelings. If the receiver suffers from skin-related issues, we might see the use of carrot seed oil or frankincense essential oil. The Carrot seed oil is an amber-colored essential oil that is extracted from carrot seeds. It's great for dry, sun-damaged, or mature wrinkled skin. Frankincense essential oil may also be used because the oil has antibacterial and anti-inflammatory properties with benefits for acne-prone skin. It is also cytophylactic. The word cytophylactic means that it helps protect existing cells and encourage new cell growth. I have witnessed that this oil helps soothe chapped dry skin.

Biblical Physicians

God's Holy Word does not record the word doctor, but instead, we can find references to physicians and healers. Biblical healers relied on the art of aromatherapy and maybe reflexology.

According to the Word in Genesis 50:2,

_____

_____

_____

Joseph commanded his servants and the physicians to embalm his father with the burial oils: and the physicians embalmed Israel. According to 2 Chronicles 16:12,

_____

_____

_____

Asa, in the thirty-ninth year of his reign, was diseased in his feet until his disease was exceeding great, yet in his disease, he sought not to the LORD but the only the earthly physicians. In Job 13:4, we find this statement,

_____

_____

_____

"But ye are forgers of lies, ye are all physicians of no value." In the word of Jeremiah 8:22, we find this statement,

_____

_____

_____

"Is there no balm in Gilead; is there no physician there? Why then is not the health of the daughter of my people recovered?" In the New Testament, we find this statement in Matthew 9:12, "But when Jesus heard that, he said unto them, they that be whole need not a physician, but they that are sick." Then, in Mark 2:17, we see a similar statement: "When Jesus heard it, he saith unto them, they that are whole have no need of the physician, but they that are sick: I came not to call the righteous, but sinners to repentance." In Mark 5:26, we find a very sick woman, and she had suffered many things from many physicians.

_____

_____

_____

"After she had spent all that she had and was nothing bettered, but rather grew worse, she sought the true physician." We find reference after reference in scripture that a physician is needed for the sick. The reference in Luke 5:31 states,

_____

_____

_____

"Jesus answered and said unto them, they that are whole need not a physician; but they that are sick." In Colossians 4:14,

_____

_____

_____

there is a reference that Luke, was a beloved physician in Demas. This explains why in his gospel recordings that he tells us of many healing miracles. The great physician is always pointing to Jesus. Physicians in the Bible days were healers that trusted their Creator. With God's directions, the healers used and prescribed essential oils from all their resources found in God's backyard. Essential oils, once again, comes from herbs, spices, and minerals God created in Genesis.

After examining three happenings in the Bible, we can conclude that after seeking modern doctors and treatments that modern medicine may not have been the best option. Today, I'm afraid that some Christians die not because they are on the prayer list, but because they did not seek our heavenly healer and simply believe. Referenced in Job 13:4,

_____

_____

_____

we find that he refuses the idea of secular medicine from his friends. Instead, Job believed God and was healed. Job 42:16 states,

_____

_____

_____

"After this Job lived one hundred and forty years, and saw his sons and his sons' sons, even four generations." In Mark 25:34 and in Luke 8:8 :43–48,

_____

_____

_____

the woman with the issue of blood was healed. This woman put her hope in modern doctors and medical treatment before God. Then, as recorded in the Bible, she touched the hem of Jesus's garment, and because of her faith, she was healed. Finally, in 2 Chronicles 16:11–14,

_____

_____

_____

the king sought the council of many healers and physicians but left God out. In addition, in 2 Chronicles 16:14, the Bible records his death and the use of essential oils for his burial.

_____

_____

_____

We need to follow the scripture found in Matthew 6:33 (KJV) that states, "Jesus said, 'Seek ye first the kingdom of God, and his righteousness; and all these things shall be added unto you.'" In conclusion, Jesus was warning us not to worry about our human concerns but, instead, place our greatest priority on seeking God's Kingdom.

Name that Physician? Be creative! It's just for fun!
Who heals with the heart, with love, with knowledge, etc.

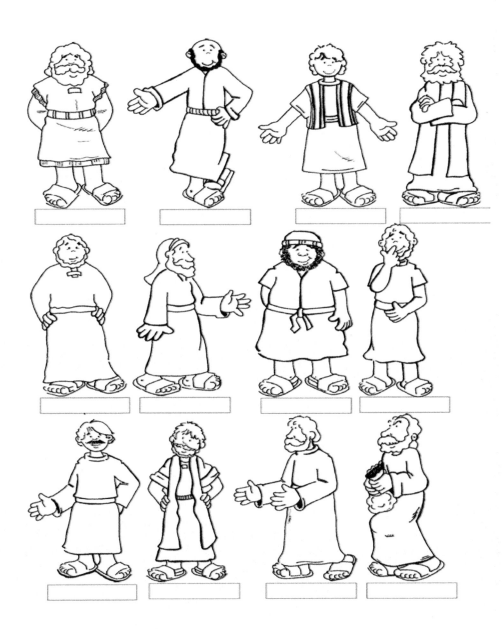

Class One:
The evidence of oil in Scripture

The answers to the following essential oil will be delivered in class.

If you are currently using essential oils jot down their usage. You may also write down a question or two.

Peppermint:

_____

_____

_____

Lemon:

_____

_____

_____

Orange:

_____

_____

_____

Emotional Blend:

_____

_____

_____

On guard:

_____

_____

_____

Sandalwood:

_____

_____

_____

Cassia:

_____

_____

_____

Cypress:

_____

_____

_____

Frankincense:

_____

_____

_____

King Solomon was a very rich king. Solomon ruled over all the kingdoms from the Euphrates River to Philistines and as far as the border of Egypt. He had an abundance of resources. He enjoyed his gardens and utilized them in his romantic endeavors. But he was now wanting to build a church for God, using the most costly, hard to get trees. He had all the riches at that time and could afford the cost. My favorite class to teach is the lesson on Cedar trees. The lessons on Cedar trees are in my next edition. Below is a map of King Solomon's property:

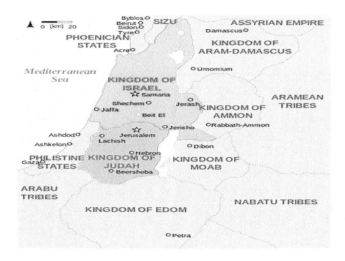

Second Chronicles 2:16 reinforces the treaty Solomon had with his worker, Huram.

_____

_____

_____

King Huram displays respect for Solomon. This verse tells us that the King was yearning to serve King Solomon. The two kings approved a deal for the timber. It was decided that the timber would delivered to Joppa, and then from there, the timber would be brought by boat. King Huram declared his dependence on King Solomon for skilled workmen.

The map below will help you visualize the exporting route of the Cedar timber.

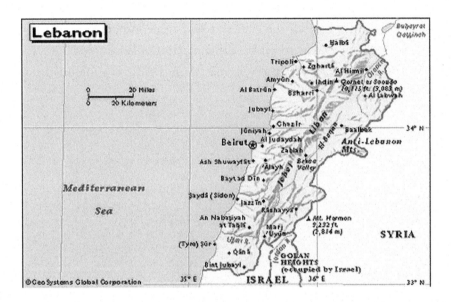

Scripture Opportunity One:

1.   Does scripture support the use of essential oil?

Isaiah 40:12

_____

_____

_____

Isaiah 40:12 contains questions not meant for us to answer but, instead, shares the notion that our God is larger than the earth. His infinite ability and power is able to control the world, but also, his divine power is able to solve the simplest problem. God is literally able to do all things. Isaiah is portraying our Sovereign God has one with all the wisdom and we are weak and our idols are foolishness. Therefore, the prophet suggests that God's divine counsel is perfect and our carnal judgment does not compare to God. In Job 28:25, this type of questioning is also weighted-out.

2.   Essential oils are in the pages of God's word.

There are over 126 plant families in the Holy Bible. Archaeologists have found plants in dig sites. The Dead Sea caverns were covered in garlic, leeks, onions, pomegranates, and a selection dates. Garlic leaves have also been discovered in Egyptian tombs. If we scrutinize God's creation, we can find figs, olive trees, and pomegranates in California. A quantity of olive trees also grows in Florida. Finally, if we look at God's colder climates, we'll find other varieties of plants, herbs, and vegetation.

Exodus 30:34–35

_____

_____

_____

At this time in biblical history, the Israelites were motionless in the desert. They were traveling to the Promised Land when the Lord commanded Moses to construct the holy anointing oil and incense. The anointing oil was used for consecrating the high priest and his sons, the altar, the Ark of the Covenant, and the tent meetings. The High Priest at this time would have been Aaron. Finally, in accordance to God's instructions, Aaron offered the fragrant incense formulated in Exodus 30:34–35 on the altar every morning and evening.

3. What did God's people report about essential oils in the Old Testament?

Proverbs 21:20 and 2 Kings 20:13

_____

_____

_____

This is the verse that provides an example of someone who is very proud of his or her possessions. Nothing is really wrong with wealth or owning treasures, but it becomes sin when we lay all our belongings in front of some to receive their approval or to show our power. We are nothing and have nothing of any worth if we do not have God. King Hezekiah had just split from the King of Assyria and was chastened by God.

4. Locate the use of essential oils in the New Testament.

Mark 14:3–9

_____

_____

_____

The Sanhedrin plans Christ's death. The woman brought oils to anoint Jesus before his death. The Passover was conducted just a couple days later. Then we read about Judas getting money to betray Jesus. This topic is covered, in detail, in the lesson of Anointing Jesus.

5.   Holistic Physicians VS. Modern Physicians

_____

_____

_____

Our current medical field is very atheistic. In school, doctors are taught nothing about God's Word. Since, modern medicine is manmade they have dangerous side effects and dependency issues. I have found no reports that someone has ever died using oils topically. The point here is that essential oils are a gift from God.

Name three benefits you want to see from using God's medicine?

_____

_____

_____

Below is a list of concerns from one of my large classes. Highlight the ones that interest you and circle one or two to share with a family member.

1.   *Anxiety:* Lavender, cedarwood is well known for being calming, but it also helps with cuts and bruises, headache, and to get more sleep.
2.   *Depression:* Peppermint elevates mood but also gets rid of nausea and congestion.
3.   Head/body ache: Lemon, ceadarwood, frankincense, sandalwood, and tea tree. These two oils, combined together, help blemishes, cold sores, and athlete's foot. Also, anoint your four-legged friend and help keep fleas away.
4.   *Can't sleep:* Lavender, vetiver, chamomile will help you relax; spray it on your pillow at night to help you sleep.

5. *Fatigue:* Grapefruit, citrus, and orange. Also helps with jet lag, affects your breathing, and congestion. This combination is also an all-natural household cleanser.

6. *Sinus Congestion:* Lime, pine, eucalyptus, lavender, peppermint, rosemary.

7. *Mental Clarity:* Four drops of rosemary, six drops of lemon, and two drops of cypress.

8. *Weight Loss Protocol:* Thirty droplets of lime, forty-five drops of tangerine, forty-five drops of orange, seventy-five drops of grapefruit, seventy-five droplets of lemon, ten drops of peppermint. Mix in a fifteen milliliter bottle. Take in a veggie capsule. Put seven to 10 drops in the morning and three to five in the afternoon when feeling hungry.

9. *Headache Relief:* Two droplets of peppermint, one droplet of rosemary, one drop of eucalyptus, two droplets of lavender.

10. *Diarrhea:* Thyme, tea tree, lavender, eucalyptus, and lemon. Apply by massaging clockwise directly on the tummy.

Scripture Opportunities for Part Two

(This is the class member's homework)

1. Aloes/sandalwood:
1.
Five Bible References:

Psalm 45:8

_____

_____

Proverbs 7:17

_____

_____

John 19:39

_____

_____

Used in embaling, _____, and_____

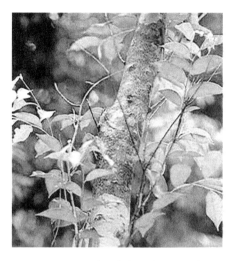

Modern Day Uses: Promotes healthy skin and emotional balance, powerful cleansing agent for mouth and throat.

2.   Cassia

Bible References:

Ex 30:24–25

_____

_____

Biblical people indemnified cassia as tropical evergreen trees with glossy, leathery leaves. The people new this evergreen could only survive in hot humid temperatures and could be forty feet tall. What buildings do you know that are forty feet tall?

Psalm 45:8

_____

_____

Cassia is the inner bark of an ever green tree (Cinnamomum cassia), which differs from that which produces cinnamon. Cassia is very fragrant, and God's people used it in perfumes.

This perfume pleasant aroma was also great to use on their garments for antifungal protection.

Biblically used in the sacred and _____ holy anointing oil given to Moses and is a _____.

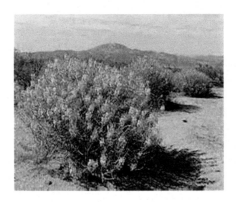

Modern Day Uses: supports healthy immune function and digestion, helps promote circulation.

3.   Cedarwood

Sixty-nine Bible References:

First Kings 5:6–10

_____

_____

First Kings 9:11

_____

_____

Second Chronicles 2:16

_____

_____

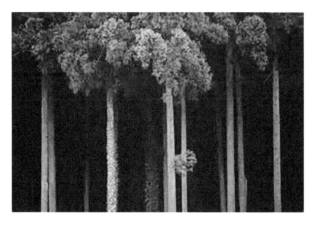

Used in purification rites and building material.

Modern Day Uses: supports healthy respiratory functions; promotes clear, healthy skin; relaxing aroma.

4.   Cypress

Twenty-four Bible References:

Isaiah 44:14

_____

_____

Isaiah 60:13

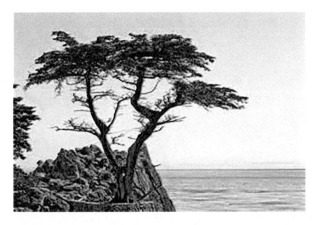

Used in purification rites, weaponry, and as building material.

Modern day uses: Promotes healthy skin, uplifts mood, promotes healthy respiratory functions, soothes tight muscles, supports localized blood flow.

5.   Frankincense

Sixty-nine Bible References:

Exodus 30:34

Matthew 2:11

Used in incense and offerings a gift given to Jesus from the Magi, was used to treat leprosy.

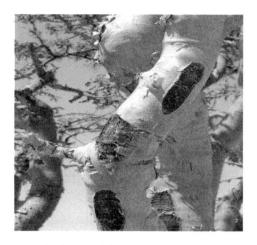

Modern Day Uses: helps build and maintain healthy immune system, promotes cellular health, rejuvenates skin.

6.   Myrrh

Bible References:

Myrrh is an expensive product that it is used for producing perfume, amalgamation of medicine and preparing incense. In sacred times, myrrh was a significant trade item. The scriptural people acquired myrrh from Arabia, Abyssinia, and India.

Exodus 30:24

_____

_____

Esther 2:12

_____

_____

Matthew 2:11

Song of Solomon 1:13

Key Information: In ancient writings, the scribes recorded myrrh being used a jewelry. Women in those days strung myrrh rocks into a necklace. The necklace was worn around the woman's neck. Egyptian women then attached a flask to the base of their necklace and created a pendant. The pendant was opened when needed to treat medical conditions like hemorrhoids and eye infections.

John 19:39

Used in incense and offerings a gift given to Jesus from the Magi, used as preservatives for oil mixtures.

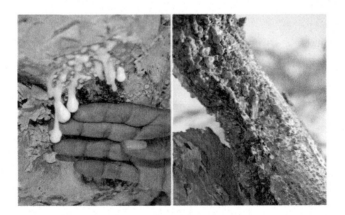

Modern Day Uses: Promotes healthy skin and emotional balance, powerful cleansing agent for mouth and throat.

Scriptural Challenge for Lesson One.

First Time student: Simply read the verse and write a key phrase about the use of oil.

Pre-qualified students: Do the work of the first time student, plus describe the verse in your own words.

Qualified Students: Do the work of the first time student and the pre-qualified student; record the verse on the lines provided from two versions: KJV and NIV. Note any differences.

Psalm 45:8

_____

_____

_____

Proverbs 7:17

_____

_____

_____

John 19:39

_____

_____

_____

Exodus 30:2–25

_____

_____

_____

First Kings 5:6–10

_____

_____

_____

First Kings 9:11

_____

_____

_____

Second Chronicles 2:16

_____

_____

_____

Isaiah 44:14

_____

_____

_____

Isaiah 60:13

_____

_____

_____

Esther 2:12

_____

_____

_____

Isaiah 40:12

_____

_____

_____

Exodus 30:34–35

_____

_____

_____

Proverbs 21:20

_____

_____

_____

Second Kings 20:13

_____

_____

_____

Genesis 1:11–12

_____

_____

_____

Exodus 30:23

_____

_____

_____

Mark 14:3–9

_____

_____

_____

Class One

Hand-Out One

Is. 40:12 (If these are not my own work, the credit is given on the image) I thank www.bling.com.

Peppermint

headache
fever
hot flashes
stomach ache
memory
nausea
shock
increase oxygen

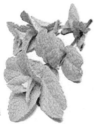

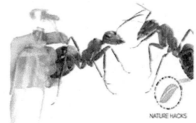

Peppermint Usage:

1. Arouses your physique

    Placing a few drops of peppermint essential oil around the tip of your nose will send a message to the brain to wake up. Incorporate peppermint essential oil in your body butter or lip balm.

2. Enhances the stomach production

    Apply a few drops to the top of your belly and massage into the skin.

3. Acts as breath mint

Peppermint essential oil is a really effective substitute for a breath mint

4. After lunch pick-me-up

Add one drop to an eight-ounce glass of water, defuse, or put one droplet under your tongue.

5. Scrub Cleaner

Add essential oil to baking soda and scrub it on the tub. Best of all, its nontoxic.

Class Two: Creation

I found the word *oil* in scripture over 640 times in the Bible. The Bible is God's Holy Word; therefore, it is not a science text that catalogs oils, herbs, and plants, but instead, the Bible is a spiritual living word that provides guidance for us to use in our lives. The Bible does directly provide a reference for which essential oil are named. Most Bible connections, however, are indirect and do not state the exact name of the plant or oils because essential oils were used by the people daily. Every biblical family owned, combined, and utilized essential oils. The next pages are to be completed in class.

How would you describe God's creation? I refer to God's creation as his backyard. Who has the verse in Isaiah 40:12? "Who has measured the waters in the hollow of his hand, or with the breadth of his hand marked off the heavens? Who has held the dust of the earth in a basket, or weighed the mountains on the scales and the hills in a balance?" And Matthew 5:35: "Nor by the earth; for it is his footstool: neither by Jerusalem; for it is the city of the great King."

In 40:12, God melted out heaven with the span. "I think of all the galaxy and stars. And comprehended the dust of Earth in a measure. He knew where to put the sand. He knew where the dirt needed to go. And even the red clay mud. He weighted the mountains in a scale. Mountains form a barrier, belt, or system that contains geological features a region." Scientists have divide the mountains into segments. For example, some mountain ranges are divided into highland, mountain passes, and valleys. For instance, I live in the application mountains, but if you live in New Hampshire, you live on in the Blue Ridge mountains.

Class Two Organizer

Creation: Bible study Two
Creation: God's Anointed Blend

Psalm 104:5

_____

_____

_____

Isaiah 40:12

_____

_____

_____

Job 34:12

_____

_____

_____

Genesis 1:1

_____

_____

_____

Proverbs 30:4

_____

_____

_____

Jeremiah 10:12

_____

_____

_____

Job 38:4–6

_____

_____

_____

Class Two: Thought Organizer in Student's Book

Menu

WHO OWNS THE WORLD? Who owns the world? WHO OWNS THE WORLD

John 1:1

_____

_____

_____

Genesis 1: 1–13

_____

_____

_____

Matthew 24:7

_____

_____

_____

Luke 21:11

_____

_____

_____

This chapter makes essential oils special. "In the beginning was the word and the word was with God and the word was God." Thus, begins the Gospel of Saint John. The creation occurrences in Genesis 1:1 begins with this statement: "In the beginning, God created the heavens and the earth." Following that, we find God speaking every-thing into existence by his Word. So God said let there be light and firmament then God sys bring forth grass, herbs, and fruit trees. We find the word, *Word*, written nine times in the scripture. The mean-ing of the word, *word*, is said to be a vibration, a frequency, and an expression of energy. God created the plants by simply speaking his *word*. God's Word includes the plants, their oils, gums, and resins. Such plants are divinely ordained form creation. Gods' instruction book prepares us in utilization of the plants for medicines. Therefore, when we need healing, the application of payer and the consumption of essential oils functions as clean health benefits for our commu-nities. Thus, this generates the notion that essential oils are crucial. They contain power from God's Word. Artificial medicine does not have such power. We can tap into God's power in prayer from the Holy Spirit. So then, why can we not cure our elements of illness?

Two scriptures come to mind: Matthew 24:7 and Luke 21:11.

"Nation will rise against nation, and kingdom against king-dom. There will be famines and earthquakes in various places" (Matt. 24:7).

"There will be great earthquakes, famines and pestilences in various places, and fearful events and great signs from heaven" (Luke 21:11).

The scripture says in the last days, pestilence will come. The definition of pestilence is that it's a contagious or infection epidemic disease. These diseases are devastating and destructive. When this happens, the Bible says the Lord's coming back.

Who knows what I mean?

_____

_____

_____

Some modern-day pestilence to discuss are as follows (www. bing.com):

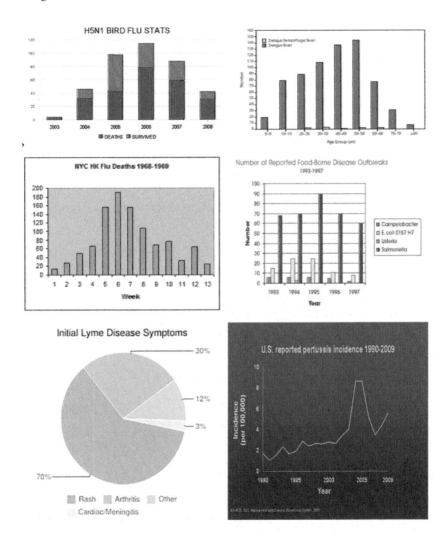

Class Two: Scriptural Challenge

First-time student: Simply read the verse and record it here as it is written in the Bible.

Pre-qualified students: Do the work of the first-time student, plus describe the verse in your own words.

Qualified Students: Do the work of the first-time student and the pre-qualified student, plus cross-reference the scriptures.

Psalm 104:5

_____

_____

_____

Isaiah 40:12

_____

_____

_____

Job 34:12

_____

_____

_____

Genesis 1:1

_____

_____

_____

Proverbs 30:4

_____

_____

_____

Jeremiah 10:12

_____

_____

_____

Job 38:4–6

_____

_____

_____

This Map shows the surrounding area of Israel.
In biblical times, all of these countries used essential oils extensively.

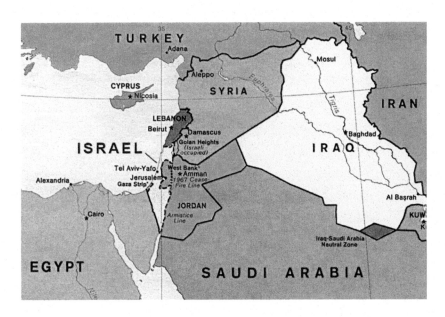

Class Three:
Health Issues that Matter!

In this section, we simply describe aging according to the Bible but then offer questions and answers to some of the most common questions people ask their wellness advocate. This class is titled as follows: Health Issues that Matter!

The Bible presents growing old as a normal part of life. According to the scriptures, there is honor in growing old. Humans can find honor because growing old is usually accompanied with an increase of wisdom. For example, when we physically get gray hair, the Bible says gray hair is a crown of splendor, and it's attained by a righteous life (Prov. 16:31, Prov. 20:29). God wants us to remember that life is short (James 4:14) and that the beauty of our youth is soon gone (Prov. 31:30, 1 Pet. 1:24). In addition, we should use our abilities to serve Christ. Once we discover God's vision for our lives, we should obey his voice. We find true happiness, living God's purpose (Jer. 29:11). Following God's mission is what makes life's experiences enjoyable. All our God-given talents and opportunities in life will soon cease. So before all your opportunities to use your gifts are gone, be sure to seize every moment (Eccles. 9:7–10, 11:9, 12:7).

In today's world, many of our older church members have become shut-ins. Shut-ins are the sickly ones that are often forgotten by the elders. However, everyone is responsible, but it seems that we still forget to visit them. Unfortunately, we do exactly what Psalm

71:9 describes: "Do not cast me off in the time of old age; forsake me not when my strength is spent." The Bible says the seniors have the most important job. Their job is to educate the youth of the church. God's Word in Psalm 92:12–15 states, "The righteous flourish like the palm tree and grow like a cedar in Lebanon. They are planted in the house of the LORD; they flourish in the courts of our God. They still bear fruit in old age; they are ever full of sap and green, to declare that the LORD is upright; he is my rock, and there is no unrighteousness in him." In the scripture, Psalm 71:18 (ESV) states, "Take heed and realize even though we are of old age and have gray hairs; Our God, will not forsake us." We should proclaim God's power to the next generation and to those to come. This leads us to understand 2 Corinthians 4:16 (ESV): "So we do not lose heart. Though our outer self is wasting away our inner self is being renewed day by day." Finally, the elderly is valuable and serve a unique and useful purpose in the kingdom.

God's Word in Psalm 92:12–15 it states, "The righteous flourish like the palm tree and grow like a cedar in Lebanon. They are planted in the house of the LORD; they flourish in the courts of our God. They still bear fruit in old age; they are ever full of sap and green, to declare that the LORD is upright; he is my rock, and there is no unrighteousness in him." Even though most of our society believe a nursing home is the way to go when you retire, God's Word says in Psalm 92:14, "They are able to bear much fruit and remain fresh in the mind and flourishing, despite their age."

Let's look at a few verses (Record them on the lines that follow the scriptures. This will help you connect to the Word).

Exodus 7:7

———————————————————————————

———————————————————————————

———————————————————————————

Psalm 90:10

_____

_____

_____

Josh 24:29

_____

_____

_____

Josh 14:6–11

_____

_____

_____

Daniel 1:21

_____

_____

_____

Daniel 6:1–3

_____

_____

_____

Daniel 6:27

_____

_____

_____

Daniel 6:28

_____

_____

_____

Aaron and Moses did extraordinary things in their own age. God chose them to lead Israel out of Egypt. Their ages were around eighty-three. Recorded in Psalm 90:10 83 would have been past the normal life span. How about Joshua and Caleb? Joshua was responsible to God for the conquest of Canaan, and he live to be well over one hundred years old

Daniel was still laboring in the will of God. He served God all the years of his life. God allowed him to live to the ripe age of seventy years old. Daniel was a governor of Babylon, and he prospered in the reign of Darius. Do not lose heart if you are aging; you still a purpose, and I challenge you to go fill it!

In the scripture, Psalm 71:18 (ESV) states, "Take heed and realize even though we are of old age and have gray hairs; Our God, will not forsake us." We should proclaim God's power to the next generation and to those to come. This leads us to understand 2 Corinthians 4:16 (ESV): "So we do not lose heart. Though our outer self is wasting away our inner self is being renewed day by day." Finally, the elderly is so valuable their unique service edifies the church. The elderly of society is useful and has purpose in the kingdom of God.

According to Acts 14:23, Titus 1:5–9, and 1 Peter 5:1–4, in God's design of the church, the elders are supposed to oversee the church's endeavors. In 1 Peter, we can read the testimony of elders of the church performing the act of being oversees. In the lines below, record the scriptures. This action will be nice when you come back to study. It will already be there.

Acts 14:23

_____

_____

_____

Titus 1:5–9

_____

_____

_____

First Peter 5:1–4

_____

_____

_____

The use of careful aromatherapy can be an effective instrument for several elderly patients. The practice of God's medicine complements traditional medicine and may stimulate the appetite, give more energy, and even promote relaxation. In the last decade, there has been a surge of interest in using essential oils to effect symptoms of dementia (Alzheimer's). Some studies detect lavender and lemon made in balm reduces anxieties and agitation. The patience caregivers have testified that peppermint stimulate the memory. Bergamot claims to fight depression and help sleep. Rosemary has actually been defused in a couple nursing homes, and this actually help some improve cognition and has done so for me. For example, try a droplet of peppermint in a glass of water approximately at three in the afternoon; it could possibly provide a pick-me-up. For an increased appetite, try a drop of citrus, cardamom, bergamot, or ginger. If the oil is not tolerated on the skin, try a diffusing neckless or on the collar of the patients clothing. If an insomnia illness consists, combine five drops of lavender and water into a five milligram spray bottle and anoint your pillow. Finally, if your loved one suffers from dry skin, the research instructs us to mix frankincense or lavender in a half used bottle of nonperfumed lotion. Then, apply the mixture to the infected area. Remember that some essential oils need to be diluted with clean, fresh water before applying to your loved one's skin. Some essential oil recipes include a carrier oil like coconut instead of distilled water. In addition to this advice, let the person smell any essential before they are applied.

Essential oils can help support and strengthen the systems of the body, including the immune, digestive, nervous, muscular, skeletal, respiratory, and cardiovascular. Using essential oils while you are young is a wise thing to do because if you live longer, who wants to be sickly? Seniors, however, still benefit from God's medicine too. For example, diffusing essential oils can support emotional balance and memory. Some aromatherapists recommend a hand or foot massage to provide support for their emotions. This process of massage in practice is known as a part of scientific reflexology. Reflexology is a system of massage techniques used to relieve tension and treat bodily illness. Scientist and biblical people understood the reflex points. The reflex points are on the feet, hands, and head, which are great places to anoint the body because the reflex points are linked to every part of the body. Scientist and biblical people understood the reflex points. The hand and foot messages benefit both the olfactory/limbic pathway. In addition, just a touch from another person could boost the mood of another person, thus creating emotional benefits from a caring touch. Finally, one of my favorite ways to apply essential oils is to simply mix some coconut oil with the essential oil itself and rub it on different areas of the body, according to where it works best for that particular oil. Because essentials oils are so small molecularly, they can actually be absorbed into your body through your skin. So you can get full body makeover by simply putting essential oils directly on the skin. Below, is a diagram of reflexology.

Study Opportunity: Issues that Matter

1. What essential oils help tolerate hot flashes?

_____

_____

_____

Essential oils, blended with peppermint and lemon, will help relieve hot flashes. Since essential oils go right through the skin, applying them to fatty areas of the body where hormones are manufactured and stored will create the most direct effect. Of course, any massage is itself very therapeutic. A bath is also a wonderful way to receive the benefits of these oils.

2. What essential oils help menopause?

_____

_____

_____

These essential oils include clary sage, anise, fennel, cypress, angelica, coriander, sage, and, to a lesser degree, basil.

Application: Since essential oils go right through the skin, applying them to fatty areas of the body where hormones are manufactured and stored will create the most direct effect. Fatty areas are sweat glands, scalp, soles of your feet, upper back, ankles, behind the ears, and temples.

3. What essential oils can help my hair loss?

_____

_____

_____

You can mix essential oils in your shampoo: clary sage, lavender, and melaleuca (tea tree) together for great results. They are also suitable for various organic hair masks and they may have different effect on hair condition depending on which natural ingredients you will use.

4. Are your hormones out of control?

_____

_____

_____

If you want to have more balanced hormones, personally, I recommend considering clary sage oil along with thyme oil. For men, I recommend the same essential oils, but also add five drops of sandalwood oil. You can just put a few drops on your hand and rub it on your skin.

5. What oils can improve the function of my heart?

_____

_____

_____

Use basil, rosemary, thyme, marjoram, and clove to improve general circulation. Along with marjoram and ginger, these oils also help normalize high blood pressure. As always, remember if you have sensitive skin be sure to mix it with coconut oil. Clove is an essential oil, when applied, produces a burning sensation for some people.

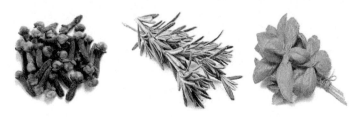

6. Is your thyroid a root of evil?

_____

_____

_____

Aromatically, diffusing precise essential oils in a diffuser (one drop of each in eight ounces of distilled water) can help energize the body. Frankincense oil also combats the fatigue and sluggishness that often times arrive with low thyroid function. Common energizing essential oils are cinnamon, eucalyptus, lemon, lime, grapefruit, rosemary, and peppermint.

7. What about PMS symptoms?

_____

_____

_____

During a woman's menstrual cycle, she feels the effects of hormonal imbalances. A number of essential oils can be used to treat the imbalances that accompany premenstrual syndrome. For example, aniseed, clary sage, fennel, and sage—all these have estrogenlike compounds that may make them effective in relieving symptoms associated with PMS.

8. Can you help me find oils to prevent hair loss?

_____

_____

_____

Essential oils have been ingredients in hair care recipes for generations. Those oils historically have been lavender, chamomile, rosemary and melaleuca (tea tree). The products have been placed in shampoos and conditioners because these oils can positively support the health of the hair follicles and scalp. These oils have been said to help the skin on your scalp open pores to absorb and provide a healthy scalp. Most shampoos and conditioners do not have all natural essential oils, and if they do, they contain only small amounts. So this is why it would be wise to add them to your personal care items, including your shampoo.

9. What might improve my acid reflux?

_____

_____

_____

Ginger essential oil comes from a ginger root. It is very common in the grocery; however, you need a therapeutic grade oil. Add two to four droplets in a hot cup of drinking water.

You may also try peppermint essential oil because it is more concentrated. Add a droplet of peppermint, a teaspoon full on apple cider, and one teaspoon of honey into a glass of water. Thirdly, try two drops of eucalyptus essential oil and three drops of peppermint in a glass of water.   Lastly, try lemon drops in water to create plain lemon water. When the water is cold, this is quite a refreshing drink.

10. Which essential oil will help a toothache?

_____

_____

_____

Try this mouth rinse: chamomile, myrrh, tea tree and peppermint. Simply add two drops warm water and wish around your mouth.

Class Two: Scriptural Challenge

First-time student: Simply read the verse and record it here as it is written in the Bible.

Pre-qualified students: Do the work of the first-time student, plus describe the verse in your own words.

Qualified Students: Do the work of the first-time student and the pre-qualified student, plus cross-reference the scriptures.

Mark 15:23

_____

_____

_____

Luke 23:56

_____

_____

_____

Luke 24:1

_____

_____

_____

Genesis 1:1–13

_____

_____

_____

Isaiah 55:13

_____

_____

_____

Exodus 30:22–25

_____

_____

_____

Deuteronomy 4:28

_____

_____

_____

Mark 15:23

_____

_____

_____

Luke 23:56

_____

_____

_____

Luke 24:1

_____

_____

_____

The chart below contains examples of some more common questions:

Complaint	Essential Oils
Stress	Lavender, lemon, bergamot, peppermint, vetiver, pine, and ylang ylang
Insomnia	Lavender, chamomile, jasmine, benzoin, sandalwood oil, sweet marjoram, and ylang ylang; lemon can wake you up
Anxiety	Lavender, bergamot, rose, clary sage, lemon, Roman, chamomile, orange, sandalwood, geranium, and pine
Depressed mood	Deep Blue, peppermint, chamomile, lavender, and jasmine
Pain	Lavender, chamomile, clary sage, juniper, eucalyptus, rosemary, peppermint, lavender,
Nausea and vomiting	Mint, ginger, lemon, orange, ginger, dill, fennel, chamomile, clary sage, and lavender
Memory and attention	Sage, peppermint, and cinnamon
Low energy	Black pepper, cardamom, cinnamon, clove, angelica, jasmine, tea tree, rosemary, sage

Lesson Three: Chart

In the section below, (use the previous two pages) simply cut and paste the complaint with the antidote. Then, when you are finished cut apart, poke a hole in the top left corner, and place each one on a key ring.

Stress	Anxiety	Pain	Nausea and vomiting
Insomnia	Depressed Mood	Memory and attention	Low energy

Black pepper, cardamom, cinnamon, clove, angelica, jasmine, tea tree, rosemary, sage	Sage, peppermint, and cinnamon	Lavender, chamomile, clary sage, juniper, eucalyptus, rosemary, peppermint, lavender,	Mint, ginger, lemon, orange, ginger, dill, fennel, chamomile, clary sage, and lavender
Deep Blue, Peppermint, chamomile, lavender, and jasmine	Lavender, Chamomile, jasmine, benzoin, rose, sandalwood oil, sweet marjoram, and ylang ylang; lemon	Lavender, lemon, bergamot, peppermint, vetiver, pine, and ylang ylang	Lavender, bergamot, rose, clary sage, lemon, Roman, chamomile, orange, sandalwood, and pine

How Essential Oils Enhance Your Well-Being

For Stress:

Lavender, lemon, bergamot, vetiver, peppermint, pine, and ylang ylang

For Low Energy:

Black pepper, cardamom, cinnamon, clove, angelica, jasmine, tea tree, rosemary, sage, and citrus

For Nausea and Vomitting:

Mint, ginger, lemon, orange, ginger, dill, fennel, chamomile, clary sage, and lavender

For Pain:

Lavender, chamomile, clary sage, juniper, eucalyptus, rosemary, peppermint, lavender, and green apple (especially for migraines)

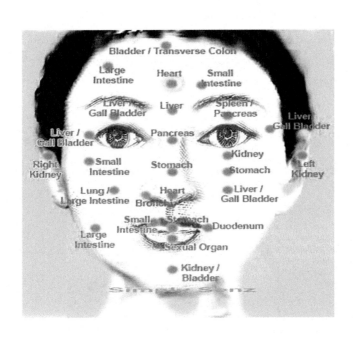

Class Three: Scriptural Challenge

First-time student: Simply read the verse and record it here as it is written in the Bible.

Pre-qualified students: Do the work of the first-time student, plus describe an example for today's world.

Qualified Students: Do the work of the first-time student and the pre-qualified student, plus cross-reference the scriptures.

1. Proverbs 16:31

_____

_____

_____

The meaning of this verse could be that if you followed the will of God all your life, you would have done much in your life. Evil would have NOT been able to lead you into sin; thus, you have lived a righteous life. The crown of glory is your reward and your honor spotlighting your persistence to do good in this world.

2. Proverbs 20:29

_____

_____

_____

This is a scripture to warn young men and old men. The Bible does not esteem one over the other; we do that! Wisdom is gained over a lifetime of learning experiences. Wisdom is the glory of the older man. The younger man's beauty is only as deep as his skin.

3. Proverbs 31:30

_____

_____

_____

It's vanity to have a countenance of beauty. The vitreous women desires to do the work of the Lord. She directs her attention toward what is profitable for the kingdom of God instead of herself. She truly fears the Lord; thus, she has wisdom and she is true to herself. She is due for the crown of glory over her life.

4. 1 Peter 1:24

_____

_____

_____

All mankind withers away like grass. The dignity, authority power, and wealth of man and women fades away. In comparison to man also the grass, very kind of herb, plants, and stalks of flowers also fade away. After death, only God's Word with exist. Only his Word will continue to be effective on earth. So spend your time wisely.

5. Ecclesiastes 9:7–10

_____

_____

_____

King Solomon, on his deathbed, late in his age, warns the young people that there is a price to pay if you give into your pleasures. At the end of your life; you can reflect on what you did and what you should have not done. The advice of this scripture is to work to make everything good in you and around you because God has a record book of your rights and your wrongs. At the end of life, there are only two choices heaven or hell. What you do in this life affects your next enteral life. Be careful; everything you do will be judged by God the Father.

6. Ecclesiastes 11:9, 12:7

_____

_____

_____

While we are young, we should be seeking the kingdom of God. We should be about our Father's business. Everyone should find God, repent, and forgive before we grow in old age. We need to seize this opportunity while we are young. Have you heard this phrase: "Don't put off today what you can do tomorrow"? Consider it! When the hour of death comes, will our thoughts be driven with infirmities or will have peace from sin?

7. 2 Timothy 5:1–2

_____

_____

_____

This scripture desires Christians to shun wrong doers of wickedness. Christians should abstain from sin. That's hard to do when shame/sin is brought into the assembly. For this reason, we must walk uprightly. In this case, a scandalous person was magnified. But instead of shunning this person, the biblical people still followed him. This man was said to be a wild scientist at that time. The Corinthians were in love with learning. In particular, they were obsessed with science and new discoveries. There thoughts height esteemed this man of science. We need to help our falling brothers, mourn for them, and not puff them up. How would you want to be treated? In our youth, we would to be absorbed in pride but in the final hours (of old age) our minds will be full of infirmities.

8. Titus 2 1–3:

_____

_____

_____

Titus is reminded his assembly on four crucial points of being a Christlike. He teaches the in truth. He tells them, man and woman, what to do and what not to do. He teaches the slaves to be obedient unto their masters. He reinitiates God's reliable measure of grace. Finally, he reminds this assembly to be consistent in their conduct.

Record additional scriptures mentioned in class. Record your addition thoughts and discoveries.

_____

_____

_____

_____

_____

_____

_____

_____

_____

_____

Class 4:
The Balm of Gilead

Map   Cottonwood Tree

Buds   Examples

Explainaton of the previous page. The products recommended may improve your health and may be utilized in place of the Balm of Gilead. Images are from www.bing.com.

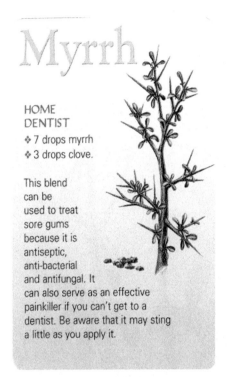

Myrrh

HOME DENTIST
❖ 7 drops myrrh
❖ 3 drops clove.

This blend can be used to treat sore gums because it is antiseptic, anti-bacterial and antifungal. It can also serve as an effective painkiller if you can't get to a dentist. Be aware that it may sting a little as you apply it.

Myrrh

immune support
analgesic
expectorant
eczema
candida
asthma
antispasmodic
athletes foot

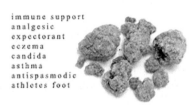

MYRRH

139 References in the Old Testament alone!

1) Apply on location for chapped lips or skin

2) Can be used topically to help break up congestion

3) Use topically on thyroid and adrenals for hypothyroidism

4) Massage into stretch marks

5) Diffuse or apply over heart for feelings of distrust or feeling unsafe

6) Use as a fixative for blends or perfumes

Blends well with: Frankincense, Lavender, Sandalwood, all Spice oils, Balance, ClaryCalm, & Whisper

First and Last Oil mentioned in the Bible!

Myrrh can directly effect the hypothalamus, pituitary, and amygdala, the seat of our emotions.

Please read the story of Joseph in its entirety before you teach or attended class this week.

In the study, pay close attention to the oils found in the scriptures. Note the scriptures and describe the details.

1.

_____

_____

_____

2.

_____

_____

_____

3.

_____

_____

_____

The first one is the most important one:
We don't claim to have all the answers, but we do know the God who does. He has all the answers and resources at his fingertips. He is a God of design, purpose, and order. Our mission and passion is to uncover the depths of the riches found in God's backyard and to suggest these findings to other Christians—hopefully, to improve the health and welfare of all!

Now for the second one, Legal requires the following:

The following statements have not been approved by the FDA. The products recommended, including the essential oils, are not intended to diagnose, treat, cure, or prevent disease. Pregnant or lactating mothers and persons with medical problems should consult their doctors.

Opening Prayer:
Father God,
We ask you, from the wealth of your glory, to give us power through your Spirit. Cast out the infirmities from our body, so we can become better and more stable laborers. We pray that we may have roots and be grounded in love. Come amongst us, Lord, and teach us today. Let the food be a nourishment unto our bodies. Bless the hands that prepared them. Amen.

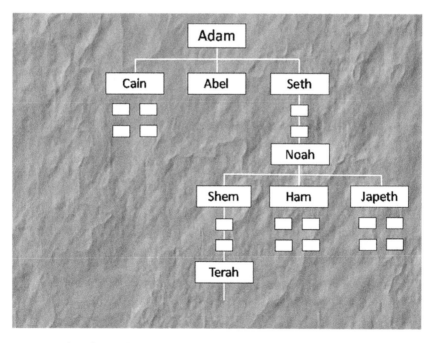

In the chart above, place Joesph where he should go. You may have to add more banches on the tree.

Please read the story of Joseph in its entirety before you teach or attend class this week.

The balm of of Gilead was actually found seven times in the Bible. Today, we can compare the cotton wood tree to the group of trees from which the balm was made from in bibical days. Cottonwood trees are a soft wood. In the spring, the wind blows, and all the dead limbs fall from the trees. The cottonwood trees contain little sticky buds. The trees grow in the Unitied States. In fact, Cottonwood trees is the state tree of Kansas has been present since 1937. They are also naturally found in Nebraska. The cottonwood tree grows to about six feet in diameter. Unfortunly, most people cut them down because the large blooms cover roofs, sidewalks, and automobiles. Most harvesters pick off the buds at the top of the tree. Native Americans burned the leaves to treat conjestion bronchitis, coughs, and whooping cough. The essential oil toned the muscle tissue and pushed out the mucus. Today, we crush the buds to create a salicylic acid. The acid is used in pain relievers.

We can harvest this either by picking off the buds from fallen limbs or by climbing the tree. Next, boil a pot of water, boil it on the stove, place the buds in a mason jar, and then place the jar in the boiling water. If you are out in the woods, you can grind the buds with your teeth or in between two rocks. Finally, place the entire crushed mixture in the wound. Cover it. This oils is said to have rapid healing powers similar to the balm of Gilead. Log onto YouTube, and search for Herbalist Yarrow Willard for a special movie clip.

The balm was renamed several times: the balm of Mecca, the balm of Jericho, and the balm of Gilead. The Hebrews said Gilead was rugged. Today, Gilead would be the land of Jordan. You can refer to the map located in the student's edition for a special reference. The land of Jordan is very mountainous and rugged indeed! The balm was first mentioned in the following:

Genesis 37:25

_____

_____

_____

Genesis 37:1–4

_____

_____

_____

When his brothers saw that their father loved him more than any of them, they hated him and could not speak a kind word to him.

Does anyone want to give us the highlights of the story?

_____

_____

_____

_____

_____

_____

_____

Joseph interpreted dreams (He was a dream catcher). Choose one dream he interpreted.

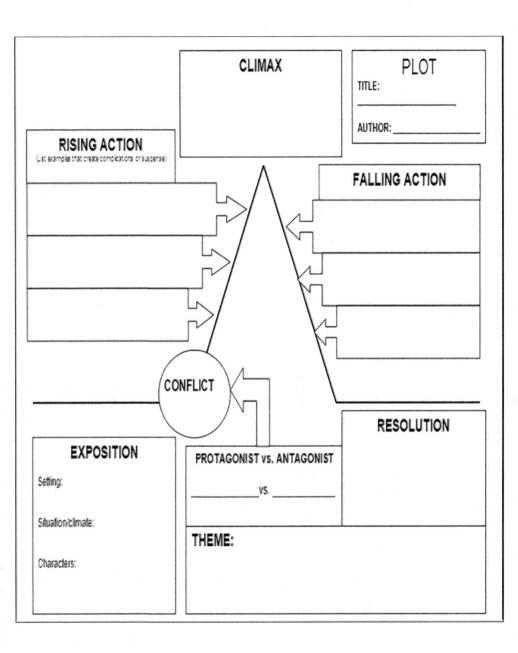

Examine all the details. Use the chart below to highlight the dream. Then, at the end of your class, ask to share your chart.

Below is an example of a dream catcher you could do with adults or children. Cut out the shapes and color. Create a circle out of a cardboard. Cover the cardboard with your favorite scrapbook paper. Make rows of braided beads and braided yarn. Cut the flowers out then layer, stacking the largest on the bottom, then the medium, and then the smallest. Remember to talk to Jesus before you go to sleep each night. You may also want to defuse serenity and lavender for deeper sleep.

Below is a picture of my dream catcher and some pictures from other class members!

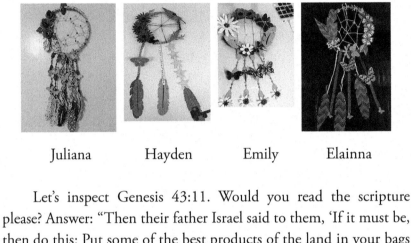

Juliana   Hayden   Emily   Elainna

Let's inspect Genesis 43:11. Would you read the scripture please? Answer: "Then their father Israel said to them, 'If it must be, then do this: Put some of the best products of the land in your bags and take them down to the man as a gift—a little balm and a little honey, some spices and myrrh, some pistachio nuts and almonds.'" In this scripture, we seen the fulfilling of Joseph's story. Jacob sent his sons to Egypt to find food. For the purpose of this class, our focus is on what the men brought and why.

_____

_____

_____

_____

_____

_____

_____

_____

In those days, the balm of Gilead would have brought a lot of money. The other oils they would have had was cassia, cedar, frankincense, myrrh, aloes (sandalwood), and cypress.

Aloes and Sandalwood

_____

_____

_____

Scriptural reference: Numbers 24:6 and John 19:39

Cassia

_____

_____

_____

Scriptural reference: Exodus 30:24 and Psalm 45:8

Cypress

_____

_____

_____

Scriptural reference: Genesis 6:14 and Isiah 41:19

Cedarwood

_____

_____

_____

Scriptural reference: Zechariah 11:1–2 and Job 40:12

The Queen of Sheba Visits King Solomon

"When the queen of Sheba heard about the fame of Solomon and his relationship to the LORD, she came to test Solomon with hard questions (v. 1). Arriving at Jerusalem with a very great caravan— with camels carrying spices, large quantities of gold, and precious stones—she came to Solomon and talked with him about all that she had on her mind (v. 2). Solomon answered all her questions; nothing was too hard for the king to explain to her (v. 3). When the queen of Sheba saw all the wisdom of Solomon and the palace he had built (v. 4), the food on his table, the seating of his officials, the attending servants in their robes, his cupbearers, and the burnt offerings he made at the temple of the LORD, she was overwhelmed (v. 5). She said to the king, "The report I heard in my own country about your achievements and your wisdom is true (v. 6). But I did not believe these things until I came and saw with my own eyes. Indeed, not even half was told me; in wisdom and wealth you have far exceeded the report I heard (v. 7). How happy your people must be! How happy your officials, who continually stand before you and hear your wisdom (v. 8)! Praise be to the LORD your God, who has delighted in you and placed you on the throne of Israel. Because of the LORD's eternal love for Israel, he has made you king to maintain justice and righteousness (v. 9).

And she gave the king 120 talents of gold, large quantities of spices, and precious stones. Never again were so many spices brought in as those the queen of Sheba gave to King Solomon (v. 10)." (1 Kings 10: 1-13)

Queen Sheba was facinated with King Solomon. In his time, everyone knew of his wisdom. His kingdom would have been holding the top rank policially. She visited King Soloman in 955 BC, according to historical dates. She saw the wonders of King Solomon's court and was even able to interview him. Upon arriving with a very great train of camels. She brought him an offering of spices, gold, precious stones, and the balm of Gilead. The balm of Gilead was not a plant that thrived in the wildrness. This tree had to be in a garden where landscapes could cultivate and harvest its oils and fruit. Queen Sheba certainly heard of King Solomons gardens, so it's reasonable to imagine she brought her crop to entice King Solomon.

Queen Sheba was the ruler of Egypt. Historically, Egypt was the first location to have the balm of Gilead, and Queen Sheba owned it. Here, in this verse, we see King Herod was in charge. He gave a direct order to have all the baby boys killed. Around that time, an angel appeared to Joesph and told him to take his family to Egypt. On the map located in the student's edition, you can see the proximaty of travel. Mary, Joesph, and Jesus were very close to the balm of Gilead trees. Thus, this brings us to the questions in your scriptural challenge. Do you think the Savior's family knew about the esssence of these trees? Do you think Jesus may have played with James under their shade? Or perhaps, Jesus and his brothers climbed the branches and picked the buds. On the other hand, was the garden gaurded and keept from our royal family with that day's royalty?

What scriptures are essential oils mentioned in the scripture?

1._____

_____

_____

_____

2._____

_____

_____

_____

3. _____

_____

_____

_____

What was the balm of Gilead?

_____

_____

_____

_____

_____

We find Queen Sheba Balquis in 1 Kings 10:10 and chapter of 11 of Chronicles.

Image from www.bing.com.

Though these five images, you can trace the existence and extinction of the balm of Gilead. I have listed them in historcial order for your convience. Be sure to label the images with the appropriate names. Use the captions for helpful hints. Record the dates of service and life.

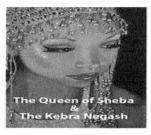

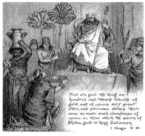

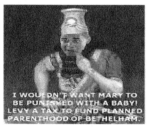

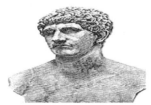

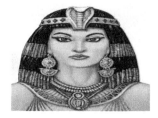

We will discuss the first three in detail. Let's read 1 Kings 10:10. Who did I assign that one to? This section will be discussed in class, but if you are overly eagar, record additional findings below:

First person:

_____

_____

_____

_____

Second person:

_____

_____

_____

_____

Third person:

_____

_____

_____

_____

Fourth person:

_____

_____

_____

_____

Fifth person:

_____

_____

_____

_____

Lastly, let's present Jeremiah 8:20, 9:1. Who did I assign this scripture to? In this scripture, we can conclude three refusals of why they did not turn back to God. In verse 4 and 7, the people refused and would not trust God. In verse 8, the people were just not wise. In the last verses, this generation, much like today, forgot not to use good jugement; and still, they did not turn back to God. Jeremiah shattered the polar view for the people that they could do what they wanted but come to the temple for protection on the Sabbath. God told Jeremiah to tell the church that was not really true. Just because you are in the room does not mean your in the right relationship with God. Jeremiah says the harvest is coming. He reminds the people the seasons have passed. Then, he questions, "How many summers must come and go before you get right with God?" With the spiritual mind he says, "Is there no balm in Gilead?" I adventure to ask: Is there no balm in the Unitied States? Is there no physician there? No healing? Where is God?

_____

_____

_____

_____

_____

_____

Help for Swollen Feet	Cleansing Foot Soak
• Two drops of lemongrass, grapefruit, and cypress. • Mix in one tablespoon of coconut oil. • Message into skin. • Fill a bowl with water and rocks. • Roll your feet back and forth. • This should help your circulation.	• One cup of Dead Sea salts • Two drops of lavender essential oil • Two drops of chamomile essential oil • Two drops of eucalyptus essential oil • Combine in a foot spa and sole
Cracked Heels	Smelling Feet
• Combine one packet or one cup of oatmeal dry mix • One cup of cornmeal • One-fourth cup of Dead Sea beads • One teaspoon of peppermint essential oil	• Tea Tree x two essential oil • Grapefruit x two essential oil • Rosemary x two essential oil • Great for antiparasitices, antifungal, antibacterial, and antiviral

Feet Fungus	Foot Pain
• Ten milliliters of roller-bottle • Twenty drops of oregano essential oil • Twenty drops of geranium essential oil • Twenty drops of melalecua essential oil • Fractional coconut oil	Hot water add: • Two drops of peppermint essential oil • Two drops of eucalyptus essential oil • Two drops of rosemary essential oil • Soak for about ten minutes.
Swollen feet	Feet Blisters
• Put one ounce of melted or fractionated coconut oil in a small jar. • Add three drops of eucalyptus essential oil • Three drops of peppermint essential oil • Three droplets of lemon essential oil	• Mix lavender essential oil and chamomile in fractionated cococnut oil and rub on feet twice a day. • Others that help are tea tree, myrrh, and geranium.

As you study with your team members and as you discuss this section in class record some thoughts about the scriptures.

Then they sat down to eat a meal. And as they raised their eyes and looked, behold, a caravan of Ishmaelites was coming from Gilead, with their camels bearing aromatic gum and balm and myrrh, on their way to bring them down to Egypt.
— Genesis 37:25 (NASB)

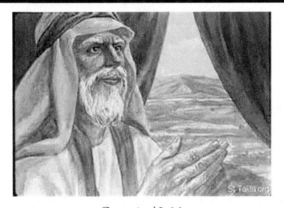

Genesis 43:11

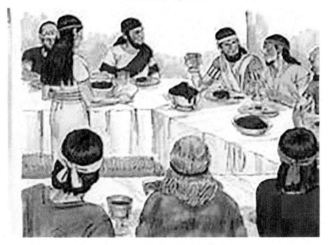

1 Kings 10:10

FLIGHT INTO EGYPT

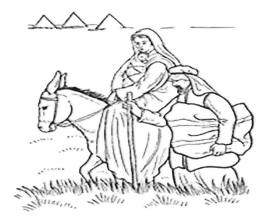

Then God sent an angel to tell Joseph to flee to Egypt
with Mary and Jesus. There they were safe.

Additional Thoughts (You will be instructed to complete this section in class.):

_____

_____

_____

_____

_____

_____

_____

_____

_____

_____

_____

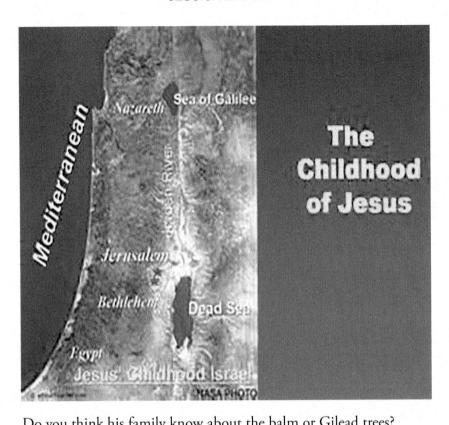

Do you think his family know about the balm or Gilead trees?

_____

_____

_____

_____

Where was the balm of Gilead when Jesus was young?

_____

_____

_____

_____

The following scriptures are in the student's guide. Put these verses on a dry-erase or black board

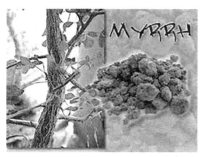
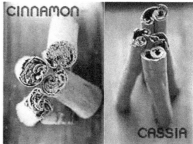

A Place for Notes—the Best Way to Study!

What is the balm of Gilead?

_____

_____

_____

_____

Joseph—Character traits:

_____

_____

_____

_____

Joseph—Story:

_____

_____

_____

_____

The scriptures:

Genesis 37:25

_____

_____

_____

Genesis 43:11

_____

_____

_____

The oils of trade:

_____

_____

_____

Oil Facts:
Sandalwood:

_____

_____

_____

Cassia:

_____

_____

_____

Cypres:

_____

_____

_____

Jeremiah 8:20, 9:1

_____

_____

_____

Shocked _____ not shocked_____ and what did Jeremiah preach?

Is it different today?

_____

_____

Does God change?

_____

Scripture _____

_____

_____

_____

_____

_____

_____

Class Five:
The Power of Anointing

Example of an Anointing Prayer for the Sick (according to www.catholiconline.com):

1. Dear Jesus, Divine Physician and Healer of the sick, we turn to you in this time of illness. O, dearest comforter of the troubled, alleviate our worry and sorrow with your gentle love and grant us the grace and strength to accept this burden. Dear God, we place our worries in your hands. We place our sick under your care and humbly ask that you restore your servant to health again. Above all, grant us the grace to acknowledge your will and know that whatever you do, you do for the love of us. Amen.

2. Lord Jesus, Lover of the sick, be with (name) in his (her) sickness. Help him (her) to accept this illness as a sharer in your cross, and bring him (her) back to full health. Lord Jesus, We praise you, for you are Lord forever and ever. Amen.

What have you learned about Exodus 30:22–25?

_____

_____

_____

_____

_____

Exodus 30:22–25

"Moreover the Lord spoke to Moses, saying (v. 22): 'Also take for yourself 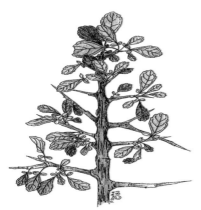 quality spices—five hundred shekels of liquid myrrh, half as much sweet-smelling cinnamon (two hundred and fifty shekels), two hundred and fifty shekels of sweet-smelling cane (v. 23), five hundred shekels of cassia, according to the shekel of the sanctuary, and a hin of olive oil (v. 24). And you shall make from these a holy anointing oil, an ointment compounded according to the art of the perfumer. It shall be a holy anointing oil (v. 25).

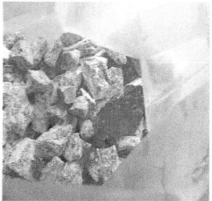

1. What is the ultimate temple in which we must worship?
Scriptures to discuss:

We must worship in a physically and spiritually clean tabernacle. Our ministers, teachers, and believers must speak the truth. We must be able to be fed with God's Word appropriately. The teachers and ministers must especially speak with clearness and be easy to understand speech. The language of the Word must be penetrated by the Holy Spirit in order to remove the veil from our hearts. If the veil covers our hearts, we can't see God. Only when Jesus rents the veil can we be saved and set free.

Luke 17:21:

_____

_____

_____

Second Corinthians 6:16

_____

_____

First Corinthians 3:16

_____

_____

_____

2. Whose duty is it to keep it clean, attractive, and in good condition?

Have you ever heard that the rocks will cry out? Christ is a living rock. We also become a living rock when Christ saves us. We should be clean and pure. Our hearts should be prepared and filled with the love for God. We should not be a stumbling rock. When masonry workers build with rock, they use the rocks that fit together. Other rocks are tossed to the side and then cause trouble. They are sharp, rough, pointed, or too vast. These are all characters of men and women who cause problems with someone else. When people pass over the stumbling block, they trip, fall, and get hurt. We need to build on the solid rock, Jesus. If we are in one mind and one accord, we will all fit and we can then build on Jesus.

First Corinthians 6:19

_____

_____

_____

First Peter 2:5

_____

_____

_____

First Peter 2:9

_____

_____

_____

Answer: According to Peter, we are all a chosen race, a royal priesthood, a holy nation, God's own people.

1. What is myrrh?

_____

_____

_____

2. What is cinnamon?

_____

_____

_____

3. What is cassia?

_____

_____

_____

4. What is ginger?

_____

_____

_____

5. What was Calamus?

_____

_____

_____

The word *calamus* is found in the KJV three times: sweet savors/ calamus in Exodus 30:23 (KJV), sweet smelling cain (NKJV), aromatic cane (ESV), and fragrant cane (NASB). Read the scriptures of Song of Solomon 4:14 and Ezekiel 27:19. In the Song of Solomon, he refers to it as a refreshing garden, and Ezekiel is speaking of cane as an export that he can sell.

Class Six:
Jesus's Earthly Anointings

Scriptural Challenge

First-time student: Simply read the verse and record it here as it is written in the Bible.

Pre-qualified students: Do the work of the first-time student plus create some notecards. On the front, put the verse title, and on the back, write out the verse. Then, ask your instructor if she or he would like to use them for class.

Qualified Students: Do the work of the first-time student and the pre-qualified student, plus cross-reference the scriptures.

1 Chronicles 9:26–30

_____

_____

_____

_____

Answer: Christians are supposed to be the leaders of worship, the leaders of offerings, and leaders of prayers

Leviticus 6:12–13

_____

_____

_____

_____

Answer: We are to be responsible for certain medical diagnoses and treatments.

Leviticus 24:2–4

_____

_____

_____

_____

Answer: We are to be responsible for certain medical diagnoses and treatments.

Chronicles 9:30

_____

_____

_____

_____

Answer: We are to care for the grounds of the church.

In the few new verses, just write the scripture in your own words. Be sure to include the who and what for each verse.

Luke 17:21

The kingdom of God was already among the Jewish nation, and they were a part of it. The devil is unleashed and seeking whom he may desire. The return of Jesus will come like the destruction the Jews have already seen.

Benefits of
Cassia Essential Oil:

Antimicrobial   Anticoagulant
Antidepressant   Antiviral
Anti-Inflammatory   Antifungal

Common Uses: Colds, Diarrhea, Kidneys, Colic
Nausea, Rheumatism, Circulation,
Stimulte Nervous System, Libido Booster,
Immune Booster, Bacterial Infection, Candida,
Atherosclerosis, Ringworm, Flu

www.ModernEssentialOils.com

10 Health Benefits of Ginger

1. Ovarian Cancer Treatment
2. Colon Cancer Prevention
3. Morning Sickness Relief
4. Motion Sickness Emedy
5. Reduces Pain & Inflammation
6. Heartburn Relief
7. Prevention of Diabetic Nephropathy
8. Migraine Relief
9. Menstrual Cramp Relief
10. Cold & Flu Prevention

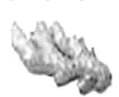

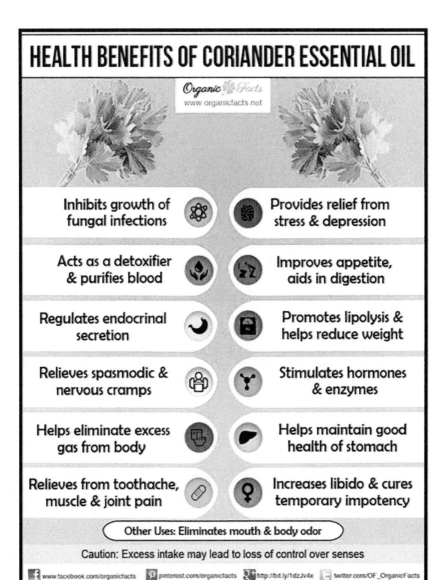

Class 6
Jesus's Earthly Anointing's
Teacher's Script

The reports of Jesus's Earthly Anointing's are often spoke about during an Easter celebration. In this study we will consider four of the gospels. I was always taught about the woman who anointed Jesus's feet; however, as I have grown older in the spirit, the Lord has lead me to understand this thought differently. I thought the account of the woman was just found in the scripture several times, but as I was lead to dig deeper, I became aware that the scriptures were different, but accurate. The woman anointed Jesus's feet and his head. Image that! Let's search the scriptures together and see if you can locate and understand each account. You are more than welcome to use the graphic organizer, class notes, and chart I've prepared in your student book.

First, read in Matt 26:1-13 in its entirety. Underline or write down if the ointment was poured on Jesus's Head or Feet?

_____

_____

_____

Secondly, read the chapter of Mark in its entirety, but focus on verses 14: 1-9. Was the ointment also poured Jesus's head?

_____

_____

_____

Thirdly, read the seventh chapter of Luke paying particular attention to verses 36-50. How was Jesus anointed in these verses?

_____

_____

_____

Then read John chapter 11. After you read this scripture come back and meditate on verses 1-2. How was Jesus anointed in these verses?

_____

_____

_____

Finally read John chapter twelve in its entirety. Then, focus on what John 12:1-8 records. Did Jesus get anointed? How?

_____

_____

_____

First, to answer the question of when accurately, investigate who wrote what and when did they write the scripture. This was very confusing for me at first glance? Since its confusing to me I included a couple graphic organizers that will help you to kept track of your thoughts.

First with this information, I started with the question, when did this account of the anointing Jesus occur?

What do you think

_____

_____

_____

_____

On the space below when did this occur per Matthew, Mark, Luke, and John?

_____

_____

_____

_____

Question One:

Two of the writers of the Bible say that the anointing occurred two days before the Passover.

Which ones?

_____

Matthew's interpretation, records this anointing took place in _____

_____.

_____ was a small village close to Jerusalem. The anointing occurred during dinner in the residence of Simon. Jesus healed Simon of his leprosy and because of his healing Simon would have been grateful to Jesus. His gratitude explains why he would have served Jesus in his dwelling. Jesus was not afraid of the germs, he didn't have to use essential oils to purify the air, Jesus brought purification with him. In final note, during a party the Children of God would burn incenses and burn essential oil to mask odors in their homes. This would have purified the air. Purification is addressed in the next addition of this book.

Mark simply states a woman. Mark's explanation, agrees that the anointing was at Simon's home, but accuses Mary the sister of Martha as being the anointer of Jesus's head. Can you visualize all the parties eating together? On the space provided describe what you have imaged?_____

Next, cooking Martha would have used fresh herbs and spices or essential oils. Today, I would same it is more common to use the fresh ingredients or dried herbs rather than essential oils. However, if you use essential oils rather than the plant leaves you only need one drop because one drop is very powerful. For example, to produce one valve of essential oil it takes several plants of oregano.

Let's switch our thinking a little. Just two decades ago it was a common practice to have the preacher and his family over for Sunday dinner. So, we can speculate what oils and spices the ladies used to cook Jesu's meal?

_____

_____

_____

If you want a more accurate estimation use a book to locate information on the best restaurants in Jerusalem and read their menu.

Did Martha glance over the dinner table at Lazarus and wonder why her sister was performing this action?

_____

_____

_____

No, she was probably in on it! Martha and Mary were sisters! Sisters devise plans together and most likely set this plan into motion. Was Lazarus and Simon sitting at the table beside Jesus?

_____

_____

_____

No doubt, all four were filled with love for Jesus. The entire evening was conducted with gratitude and was a performance of love.

Luke's description reports that the woman was from the city, but with further investigation, the women was probably also a maid-servant. Luke does not identify her name. Instead, he elaborates on the point that she was a sinner, but still does this amazing act. This description, identifies Jesus what at a civilian event with the Pharisees. The maid-servants were usually the ones hired to wash the feet, because this occupation would be considered toady as one who cleans toilets. Luke never says the lady looked Jesus in the face. She was no doubt seen as scum in her day, but Jesus saw here as a daughter of his kingdom and therefore he did not turn her away. She anointed his feet with perfumed oil and used her hair to wash his feet. As a final act of admiration, she kissed his feet. In those days, a kiss on the lips was reserved for marriage.

According to Luke 7:36-50, the Pharisees asked Jesus to dinner, in the city. The women were behind Jesus crying. Her tears ran down her face into her hair. She then washed Jesus's feet with her hair. The Pharisees got mad at Jesus' for letting this prostitute touch him. The Pharisees were so boastful that they believed "they were all that and a basket of chips too!" They thought so highly of themselves that no one should touch such a high power.

Per the book of John, the anointing of Jesus took place six days before Passover. On that day, Jesus leaves the cathedral in Jerusalem and walks about two miles to Lazarus dwelling. Jerusalem was a busy metropolitan area like our Washington D.C. Jesus was not safe sleeping any closer to the temple, because of the unbelief and malicious of the people. The family of Lazarus arranged an abundant feast for Jesus. Jesus undoubtedly loved Lazarus and his family. Jesus knew this would be his last earthly dinner with them. Mary delivered their admiration and love for Jesus by anointing him. The sweet-smelling fragrant perfume filled the interior of the homestead. This illustration is parallel to the Holy Ghost filling our sanctuary.

Also, according to Luke, the woman seems to be related to Martha. Specifically, does the scripture state who she was for sure? If so what was her name? Who was she? How many times did he refer to the woman?

_____

_____

_____

So, myrrh was in this very expensive carved box made of rock. We understand Mary and the other women had myrrh inside but what other essential oils was included? The Greek word for myrrh is *muron*. This form of myrrh was used so many times in the Bible because it was very aromatic. This form of Myrrh appears _____ times in the Gospels. Three of those times was by Matthew. Two of those were recorded in Mark. In Luke, there were four references, and four more times by John in his Gospel. For extra credit, record the references.

Matthew	Mark	Luke	John
1._____	1._____	1._____	1._____
2._____	2._____	2._____	2._____
3._____	3._____	3._____	3._____

Myrrh was used so many times, and was the most common among the Jews because it was a fixing oil. The fixing oil of myrrh was used in most oil preparations because it made the blend last longer, and it gave the aroma a boost. For example, the fragrance the Jewish used in their businesses was myrrh because it's a fixative oil that, when mixed with other oils, will fix the odors, assuring the fragrances to last longer. Myrrh is known to be one of the most effective fixing oils and has been used for thousands of years through the world. Myrrh was not only used by God's people, but also in the ancient cultures of China, India, Sumer, Babylon, Arabia, and Egypt.

It is interesting to note that myrrh is the only oil mandated by God in Exodus 30:23. It's also interesting that the thirteen times *muron* is mentioned, it is translated as ointment.

All four Gospels agree the ointment was precious because the ointment was imported and very costly. According to John's scriptures, he mentions that there was a pound of anointing oil. Today, and even in biblical times, the cost of myrrh and spikenard are both pretty high. For an accurate price, you must consider how dangerous it was to harvest and transport the plants. I believe spikenard was a bit costlier than myrrh. Today, in this twenty-first century, in American dollars, the cost of both would be around $1,000. I don't believe many of us could afford to give such a gift, but the woman did give it to Jesus. Would or could you or I do this for Jesus? To give you a better perspective, in Bible days, the amount of money would have been one year's wages.

_____

_____

_____

_____

How?

_____

_____

_____

_____

Following chart is a visual depiction of the conclusion.

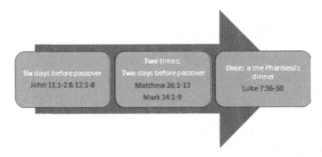

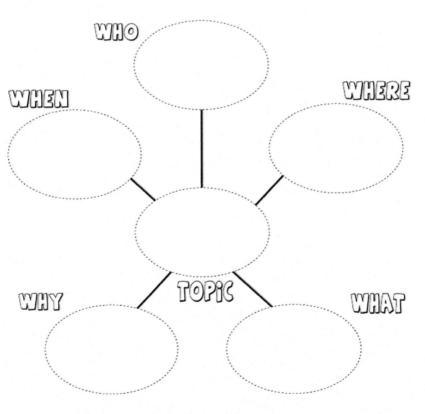

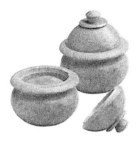

Record who, what, when, where, and how the woman anointed Jesus.

Matthew 26:1–13	Mark 14: 1–9
Luke 7 :36–50	John 11:1–2 and 12:1–8

Class notes:

When:
With this information, I started with this question: When did this account of the woman anointing Jesus occur?
What do you think?

_____

_____

_____

What:
Specifically, does the scripture state who she was for sure? If so what was her name? Who was she? How many times did he refer to the woman?

_____

_____

_____

So, Myrrh was in the box, but what else?

_____

_____

Today, in this twenty-first century, in American dollars, the cost of both would be around $1,500 to 1,000. I don't believe many of us could afford to give such a gift, but the woman did give it to Jesus. Would or could you or I do this for Jesus? To give you a better perspective, in Bible days, the amount of money would have been one year's wages.

_____

_____

_____

What conclusion can be made about the woman who anointed Jesus with essential oils?

_____

_____

_____

Below is a modern recipe for the feet. Give it a try at the end of class and talk about it! I got it from www.mydotter.com/craftryfarmer. Click on the How to tab for more recipes.

You don't have to stress about cracked heels on your feet. Try this nourishing foot mask made with doTERRA Bergamot essential oil (and other feet-friendly ingredients) for nourished and beautiful feet.

Why use a foot mask?

Since our feet have the most pores per square inch than any other area of the body, it is important to remember to treat the feet too! What you put on the feet will absorb into the rest of the body, so do your best to gather high quality, organic ingredients for this foot mask.

Ingredients:
Half cup of organic Greek yogurt
Two tablespoons of organic raw honey
Two splashes of doTERRA Fractionated Coconut Oil
One stalk of organic celery
Six drops of Bergamot essential oil

Notes about ingredients used:
- The probiotics in Greek yogurt help deliver beneficial proteins, and the lactic acid it contains rids the surface of old cells, making way for radiant, fresh skin.

- Celery is rich in zinc, which helps to repair dry, cracked skin. Celery also carries vitamins and is cleansing and detoxifying.
- Raw honey is a natural humectant, contains beneficial enzymes and antioxidants, and has antibacterial and anti-inflammatory properties.
- Bergamot essential oil is calming and soothing to the skin.

Directions:

1. Grate stalk of celery and drain excess moisture in strainer or with paper towel.
2. Add celery and remaining ingredients to food processor or blender. Blend until smooth.
3. Ready a wet washcloth or sit by tub.
4. Apply mask immediately to entire foot with fingers or brush.
5. Let sit for fifteen to twenty minutes while enjoying the mask's cooling sensation and the calming effects of Bergamot essential oil.
6. Rinse off and enjoy your nourished and moisturized feet.

See more at: http://doterra.com/US/en/blog/diy-foot-mask#sthash. BTExKE13.dpuf

Class Seven:
The Shepard/Psalm 23

Read Psalm 23 in its entirety.

This is a song written by King David. David was a shepherd by trade. So he knew full well the relationship between a shepherd and his sheep. For a moment, let's brainstorm some character traits of sheep. Record your information on your graphic organizer.

I interviewed twenty farmers in the Kanawha County Chapter of the USDA for West Virginia and several farmers I knew who were sheep shepherds. The main thing I asked them was to provide the character traits of their sheep.

I asked for good character traits and poor character traits. Therefore, the chart below will explain my conclusions.

Good Character Traits Pros	Poor Character Traits Cons
Safety in numbers	Rapid flight
Leader sheep	Stupid
Flocking together	Gullible
"Wait for me" attitude	Hogging food
Lovable	Jealous
Come when called	Getting out
Nurture their own young	Helpless
Sheep shearing and selling	Pasturing
4-H Fair and Watching them play	Weak
Feeding the babies bottles	Shearing
Livestock guarding behavior	Fainting
	Expensive
	Vet Bills
	Winter
	Confident
	Predators
	Birthing indoors

You may add your own to the list.

Recommended natural oils: chamomile, clary sage, fennel, marjoram, peppermint, rosemary, sage.

Name:_____ Date:_____

Write or draw adjectives in the ovals below that describe the noun in the middle oval.

shepherd

We should also understand that Jesus declares that he is the good shepherd, thus making him God. "I am the good shepherd: the good shepherd giveth his life for the sheep" (John 10:11). However, in this study, we want to see the characteristics of a good shepherd and how we are in the role of a sheep. In each bubble, write a trait of a good shepherd and a scripture to prove the message is correct.

What does the shepherd do for his sheep?

John 10:14

_____

_____

_____

Psalm 23:1

_____

_____

_____

Chronicles 24:15–17

_____

_____

_____

Psalm 23:2

_____

_____

_____

1 Peter 5:14

_____

_____

_____

Psalm 23:3

_____

_____

_____

Psalm 23:4

_____

_____

_____

Luke 15: 3–7

_____

_____

_____

Psalm 23:5

_____

_____

_____

1 Timothy 2:15

_____

_____

_____

Numbers 27:18–19

_____

_____

_____

Psalm 23:6

_____

_____

_____

John 10:10

_____

_____

_____

Additional shepherd characteristics from classmates:

_____

_____

_____

Write eight character traits of a Good Shepard (Based your results on responses of classmates):

1.

2.

3.

4.

5.

6.

7 and 8.

You may be asked to read Psalm 23 orally, but then, you may create a piece of photo art using the image below.

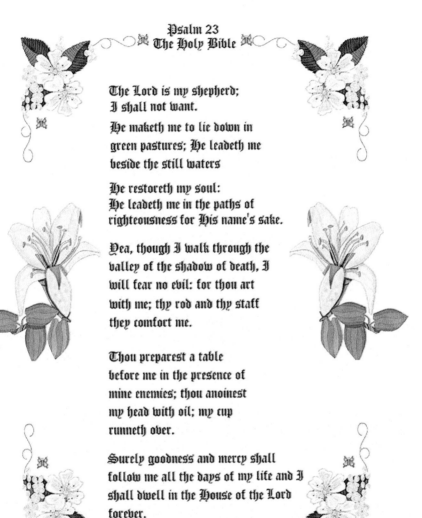

He restores my soul, He guides me in paths of righteousness for his name's sake. *Psalm 23:3*

What does the Good Shepherd do for us?

John 10;11

_____

_____

Psalm 23

Romans 7:5

_____

_____

WWW.MYDOTERRA.COM/CRAFTYFARMER

WWW.FINDINGHEALINGIN-

GODSBACKYARD.COM

Hebrews 2:1

_____

_____

You prepare a table before me in the presence of my enemies; you anoint my head with oil; my cup runs over. —Psalm 23:5

First John 2:16

_____

_____

Romans 7:5, 8:8

_____

_____

1 Sam 17:34-3

_____

_____

Matthew 24: 7

_____

_____

_____

Luke 21:11

_____

_____

_____

Psalm 23:3

_____

_____

_____

Psalm 46

_____

_____

_____

References for Psalms 23:4

The 23rd Psalm

The Lord is my shepherd, I shall not want. Psalm 23:1

```
Y   J   S   M   M   V   V   H   O   U   S   E   J   R   C
W   E   V   I   L   U   F   A   H   F   N   K   G   L   K
R   O   D   R   T   N   H   W   L   E   U   X   O   V   P
G   G   U   I   D   E   W   R   E   L   D   U   O   N   A
T   A   B   L   E   K   A   R   S   S   E   A   D   G   S
P   C   H   W   L   E   G   M   M   S   Z   Y   N   D   T
R   C   O   A   F   C   Y   X   E   T   Z   S   E   G   U
R   O   W   M   P   A   O   T   R   A   N   H   S   D   R
E   W   U   S   F   R   C   K   C   F   B   A   S   L   E
S   A   P   I   D   O   E   S   Y   F   K   D   U   W   S
T   T   U   P   Q   K   R   P   W   C   I   O   C   Y   L
O   E   T   C   A   U   B   T   A   P   S   W   L   L   L
R   R   F   V   S   T   I   F   O   R   E   V   E   R   Y
E   S   D   E   A   T   H   E   U   Y   E   W   G   Z   Z
S   E   N   E   M   I   E   S   T   A   D   J   A   E   T
```

Chapter Eight: The Sheep

Let's examine the sheep.

Matthew 5:45

_____

_____

_____

Who has Matthew 11:28?

_____

_____

_____

First Corinthians 5:5–7? What should we do?

_____

_____

_____

Hebrews 11:25. What should we do?

_____

_____

_____

Fourthly, this flock of sheep carries one another's burdens. They have one another's back. They flock together. In church, we also share one another's burdens. We come to church to be a servant to one another. We show a moment of care and affection.

Galatians 61:2

_____

_____

_____

Fifthly, when pests came, it troubled the flock and the shepherd.

Psalm 23:5

_____

_____

_____

Isaiah 41:13

_____

_____

_____

Who has John 10:28?

_____

_____

_____

Gland Relief for Opie
Formula:
Four drops of lavender
One drop of myrrh
Two drops of melaleuca
Two drops of rosemary
Two drops of eucalyptus
Tow drops of lemon
Thirty drops of Fractionated
Coconut Oil
Directions: Use a small
amount of this formula
on a make-up sponge/
washcloth. Wipe the rectum
of the dog once; at night.

Flea Be-gone!
Formula:
Eight drops of cedarwood
Four drops of lavender
Four drops of arborvitae
Fill the rest of the bottle with
distilled water!
Directions: Fill the glass
bottle with this formula!
Spray your pet once a day for a
week. Then once a week. If you
are going birdwatching, spray
your pet before you go. This
mixture can also be applied
to your clothes and body!

Patches Allergy Mixture
Formula:
30 drops of coconut oil
Severn drops of lavender
Three drops of geranium
Two drops of roman chamomile
Three drops of ylang ylang
Directions: Add this mix
into a small glass spray bottle
and spray you cat or dog
down once in the morning
and once after dinner.

Class Nine:
Rejoice with Thanksgiving

Now for the second one, Legal requires the following:
The following statements have not been approved by the FDA. dōTERRA's and other products are not intended to diagnose, treat, cure, or prevent disease. Pregnant or lactating mothers and persons with medical problems should consult their doctors.

What comes to your mind when you meditate on the word *joy*?

_____

_____

_____

What comes to your mind when you hear the word, thanksgiving?

_____

_____

_____

How are the words joy and thanksgiving alike?

_____

_____

_____

Joy from God feels like what to you? Describe joy in the space provided.

_____

_____

_____

According to the dictionary, what is the definition?

_____

_____

_____

Class Nine: Scripture Opportunity

Joy according to the world is totally different from the joy God gives to each of his children. I believe that God gives me an overwhelming sense of comfort and contentment. Joy truly floods my body and lodges deep in my soul. When we have that deep joy down in our soul, we are daily walking with the Holy Spirit. We then allow the Holy Spirit freedom to modify the deeds of our flesh (Rom. 8:13, KJV).

_____

_____

_____

According to Philippians 2:3–5 (KJV), true joy comes when we focus on the needs of others and we are obeying the directions of the Holy Spirit.

_____

_____

_____

Since joy is fruit of the Spirit, only a true follower of Christ obtains joy, and this is a special gift from God (Eph. 1:12–14, 4:30).

_____

_____

_____

Ephesians 4:30

_____

_____

_____

What comes to your mind when you meditate on the word *joy*? Are there any scriptures that enter your mind?

_____

_____

_____

According to the dictionary, what is the definition?

_____

_____

_____

Locate an event in the Bible where the Israelites found joy in God? Respond to as many as you want. If you are stuck, start with this hint: Joshua 6:1–7. Describe why the people were joyous.

_____

_____

_____

True joy from God feels like what to you? Describe joyous times in the space provided.

_____

_____

_____

In ancient cultures all over the world, people in tribes have had one person assigned to the position of healer. The healers of the tribe were also their spiritual leaders. According to God's Word, pouring on essential oils was an outward way to express joy. Let's examine the following verses of scripture:

Psalm 45:7–8, Proverbs 27:9, Isaiah 61:3, and Hebrews 1:9.

Record the verse in your own words and state what emotion is noted.

1. Psalm 45:7–8

_____

_____

_____

2. Proverbs 27:9

_____

_____

_____

3. Isaiah 61:3

_____

_____

_____

4. Hebrews 1:9

_____

_____

_____

Psalm 45:7–8

_____

_____

_____

Proverbs 27:9

_____

_____

_____

Isaiah 61:3

_____

_____

_____

Hebrews 1:9

_____

_____

_____

As we study these four verses of scripture, we notice that the names of some oils are mentioned; however, in most verses, no names are given. I think that vegetable oils may have been used as a carrier oil. I base my belief on the reports of scientists. Scientists today report essential oils to have mood-altering abilities. Vegetable oils are totally different than essential oils because veggie oils do not have the ability to stabilize our mood. Below is a list of essential oils that one considers when trying to change the status of mood. Use this sheet in class!

Confidence

_____

_____

_____

According to the Bible, the words that mean confidence is found fifty-four times in the King James Version. The Bible declares there are mechanisms and possessions that we should not place our confidence in. For example, Philippians 3:3 states, "Have no confidence in the flesh." We are deceitful people, and we even deceive ourselves. We put confidence in everything, but God. According to the scriptures, we should trust God. In reference to Psalm 118:8–9, "It is better to trust in the Lord than to put confidence in man." Can we even count the number of times man has let us down?

Depression

_____

_____

_____

The answer for depression rests on godly joy. The Bible articulates that the Holy Spirit fills us with joy and praise (Phil. 4:4, Rom. 15:11).

Several wellness advocates in West Virginia report that creating a roller-ball remedy of lemon, orange, citrus, and grapefruit, rolled behind the ear several times a day, has lesson their depression symptoms.

Loneliness

_____

_____

_____

Look back at the class on growing old. As we get older, sometimes, we isolate ourselves. God gives us purpose (Phil. 2:13). He wants us to trust him and build a relationship with him (Prov. 35:6).

We are not alone; we have Jesus right in our very own hearts (John 16:32)

Happiness

_____

_____

_____

Psalms 37:3 speaks about watching evil doers be rewarded and even be happy, but we are to be warned that this happiness fades. Only the happiness God provides is enteral secure.

Stress Relief

_____

_____

_____

God's words and our prayer life is stress relief for Christians. Consider this verse in Philippians 4:6–7. The aptitude of this segment is just overwhelming! It states, "Be anxious for nothing, but in everything by prayer and supplication, with thanksgiving, let your requests be made known to God; and the peace of God, which surpasses all understanding, will guard your hearts and minds through Christ Jesus." Go on, read it again. Did you notice all the questions? What were they?

You're right! There is potential mentioned in this verse. The verse assures that God will endow you with tranquility. Hand over all your worries, trials, and tribulations to the Lord because he provides for you. Just ditching your problems on somebody you know will resolve them should be all the stress relief we need.

Anxiety/Fear

_____

_____

_____

Just the words in this scripture calm the fear inside me: "Fear not, for I am with you; be not dismayed, for I am your God; I will strengthen you, I will help you, I will uphold you with my righteous right hand" (Isa. 41:10, ESV). Claim this promise in prayer!

_____

_____

_____

Fatigue

_____

_____

_____

Guess what the Bible says? Read Isaiah 40:29 (ESV): "He gives power to the faint, and to him who has no might he increases strength." Consider Matthew 11:28–30 (ESV): "Come to me, all who labor and are heavy laden, and I will give you rest. Take my yoke upon you, and learn from me, for I am gentle and lowly in heart, and you will find rest for your souls. For my yoke is easy, and my burden is light." Does this quicken your heart as it does mine?

_____

_____

_____

Agitation

_____

_____

_____

If you suffer from road rage, defuse mandarin or sandalwood in your car. It is not recommended that lavender is defused in the car because lavender is an all-natural sleep aid. The Bible says to practice slow to speak and slow to anger. We find all the emotions in God's Word. God made them all, and none of them should make us feel poorly about ourselves. If we have an area of concern, we should seek the Physician above all other physicians, an earthly doctor too, and the use of essential oils—accompanied with prayer, which can produce miracles for those who believe.

Memory Boosters

_____

_____

_____

If you suffer from memory block, place a droplet of cypress on your right thumb, inhale, and watch your creative juices start to flow. According to the Bible, God provides memory. If we want more memory, anoint oneself (maybe in class) and ask for what you need. Below are three scriptures that might help you.

This question will be discussed in class: How do essential oils stimulate smell in the body? The easiest way to locate an answer is to do a web search. You may also refer to the diagram on the next page.

_____

_____

_____

How do essential oils stimulate smell in the body?

The brain is a very complex organ, but for our purpose, we will divide it into two sections, the logical chunk of the brain and the detecting portion of the brain. The logical part of the brain is placed to the front, including your forehead. The rational brain excludes the uses of the four senses, but the detecting section of the brain takes over this process. The part of the brain that uses our four senses is located in the back of the brain. So let's concentrate directly on the sense of smell. We can all agree on the fact that our nose is where the sense of smell starts. In the science world of today, the sense of smell can be easily explained in a simple process. First, we breathe in deeply. That scent travels to the back of the brain (to the detecting section) and then to the frontal lobe (logical proportion), where the smell is identified. The rational brain decides what the smell is and what to do with this information. For example, the ability to read comes from the rational brain, but when we sense a smell, that sense connects us to a memory. Then, that is the work of the detecting section. These two parts of the brain work together to store our memories.

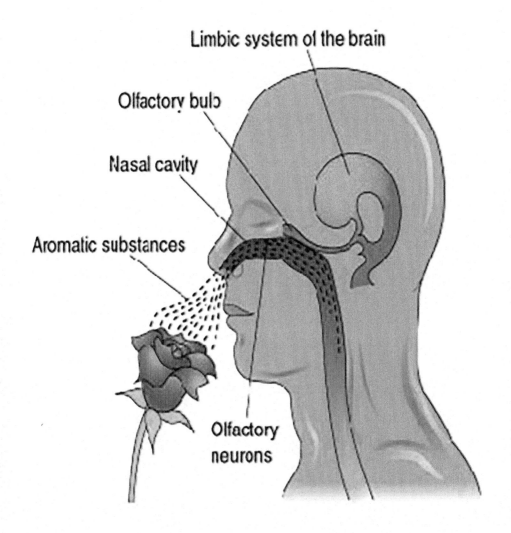

Class Ten:
Should I Take Vitamins?

"Should I take vitamins daily?" is a frequently asked question. Perhaps your physician would provide you with the best answer. I can't give you a definite answer to this question, but I did do some research. I asked ten doctors in West Virginia, "Do you suggest a multivitamin to every patient?" Most of the doctors I surveyed said they do not recommend daily vitamins to their healthy patients. Even some of the Holistic doctors surprised me with their answers. Most of the doctors agree that vitamins could be described as an insurance policy for nutrition. Finally, from my research, I'm convinced that daily vitamins are necessary.

For me, daily vitamins are a must. My fleshly body can be described as being in poor condition when considering my age. I have tried a number of vitamins off the shelf at my favorite stores, but once I tried DōTERRA's vitamins, I decided they were the most beneficial for me. After about three weeks, I noticed an increase of energy. I noticed my hair stopped falling out, and it's in the best condition than it's ever been! On my last visit, my hair stylist even congratulated me because she said whatever I am doing is working. Until now, I've never had soft, healthy hair. But the truth is in the pudding, right? When I went to my last doctor's appointment, she said this is the first time in three years that I do not need a prescription for vitamin D pills. I also have been struggling with a digestion issue (too private to record) for eight years. But thanks to God's medicine, I'm doing much better. In conclusion, all-natural vitamins have my vote.

It is not only important to feed our physical bodies, but it's also important to feed our spiritual man. So, how do the scriptures give us a daily vitamin? First, let's examine the scriptures. Let's begin with Matthew 6:11. In this verse, what does Jesus mean?

_____

_____

_____

Every word in this scripture can teach us a lesson if we stop to examine it. In this verse, we ask for bread. I believe that this teaches us to constantly depend upon Tthe Great Physician. We must be sober and patient. We don't normally seek daily bread of someone else, right? Generally, we seek God to provide what we need. It is awesome that we do not have to buy God's provisions. It's also equally great that God does not lend it to us. We are discovering in this verse that we not only seek physical food, but more immortally, we are seeking the mysteries of God's kingdom.

Next, investigate these verses and decide if the scripture is talking about spiritual food or physical food.

Ruth 1:6

_____

_____

_____

As a patient
Proverbs 30:

_____

_____

_____

Isaiah 33:16

_____

_____

_____

Luke 11:3

_____

_____

_____

So, how does the Holy Bible provide us with a daily dose of healthy vitamins?

_____

_____

_____

All Christians need to have a dialogue with Christ. However, to receive anything from God (including a daily vitamin), we must repent our sins and accept Jesus as our Lord. A daily dose of vitamins from the Bible begins with a prayer. Dialogue means to have a conversational speech with someone and, in this case, with God. The daily dose equips us to be instant in season and out of season. Second Timothy 4:2 states, "Preach the word; be instant in season, out of season; reprove, rebuke, exhort with all longsuffering and doctrine"

(Holman Christian Standard Bible). Proclaim the message. Persist in it whether convenient or not. Rebuke, correct, and encourage with great patience and teaching. Our minds are vast, but we can only build our understanding in small increments. So, why not have a daily dose?

Which type of vitamins do you need? Physical _____ or Spiritual _____

Why?

_____

_____

_____

Legally, I can't tell you what to take, and I have no training in the area of medicine. I can only suggest. So I hope this next section is helpful in your quest for good health. I ask God to grant you many healthier years.

Let's take a look at my vitamins because I am familiar with this product. I hope you can identify an all-natural vitamin versus a secular, man-made vitamin.

Examine the labels on all your vitamins bottles.

Let's look at this example (You may bring a bottle of your favorite vitamins to class for a comparison. You may use the Venn diagram located in this book, and it's about two pages from this page.):

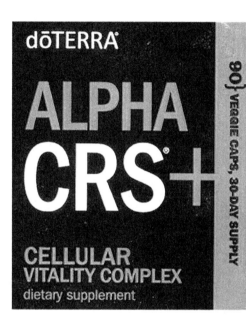

Supplement Facts

Serving Size: Three (3) Capsules
Servings per Container: 30

	Amount Per Serving	% Daily Value
Cellular Longevity Blend:	870 mg	**
WOKVEL®† Boswellia serrata (gum resin) extract (300 mg)		
Scutellaria Root extract (50 mg Baicalin)		
Milk Thistle (seed) extract (100 mg Silymarin)		
Polygonum Cuspidatum (root) extract (50 mg Resveratrol)		
Red raspberry (leaf) extract (20 mg Ellagic Acid)		
Pineapple extract (2400 GDU Bromelain protease enzyme)		
Turmeric Root extract (30 mg Curcumin)		
Grape Seed extract (20 mg Proanthocyanidins)		
Tomato Fruit extract (1 mg Lycopene)		
Marigold Flower extract (3 mg Lutein)		
Cellular Energy Blend:	410 mg	**
BACOGNIZE®† Bacopa monnieri extract (200 mg)		
Quercetin (50 mg)		
Coenzyme Q10 (50 mg)		
Alpha-Lipoic Acid (50 mg)		
Acetyl-L-Carnitine (50 mg)		
dōTERRA Tummy Tamer™ Blend:	30 mg	**
Peppermint Leaf, Ginger (root) powder,		
Caraway Seed		

** Daily Value not established.

Other Ingredients: Vegetable hypromellose, vegetable fatty acid, silica.

Directions: Adults, take 3 capsules per day, with food.

Note: Keep out of reach of children. Pregnant or lactating women and people with known medical conditions should consult a physician before using. Do not use if safety seal is broken or missing. Does not contain milk or wheat products. Store in a cool, dry place. Manufactured in the U.S.A. exclusively for dōTERRA Intl, LLC, Orem, UT 84057

† Registered trademarks of Verdure Sciences, Inc.

* These statements have not been evaluated by the Food and Drug Administration. This product is not intended to diagnose, treat, cure, or prevent disease.

dōTERRA's Alpha CRS+ is a proprietary formula of food-derived ingredients combining potent levels of powerful polyphenols and standardized botanical extracts that support healthy cell proliferation and lifespan with important metabolic factors of cellular energy.* Alpha CRS+ is formulated to be used daily with xEO Mega® and Microplex VMz™ as a comprehensive dietary supplement foundation for a lifetime of vitality and wellness. (Made with HPMC vegetable capsules.)

The first thing that I noticed on the label was the oil blend I was mixing for myself every morning. My recipe was as follows: peppermint, ginger, and parsley. This blend is known as the tummy tamer. I thought the pills from my weight loss center were the best. Now, I consider them to be good but not the best. I was concerned about the cost, but these vitamins are worth the increase in price. Let's examine some of the other good things we see on the label. This label reveals great details. When you are shopping for vitamins, the description of ingredients is the most important idea on the label. Another thing we should see are the directions and dosage. Thirdly, I actually research any unknown words to me from the label. For example, the words caraway seed was foreign to me, but they are seeds found in the parsley family. This product includes features like botanical extracts, carotenoids, and polyphenols. Finally, consider the health statement. On this label, it claims to help improve the lifespan of the consumer. This label also states that the supplement will increase cell proliferation. Well, can I really prove that? Probably not, but after consuming this product, I did have more energy, and my immune function seems to be working properly.

What did we miss?

_____

_____

_____

Record what you would like to share with the group.

_____

_____

_____

If you do take vitamins, compare the labels. If you can do that, then you have reached the goal of this class!

For homework, grab a couple vitamins you take. Below is a chart that depicts what you should notice on your label. You want

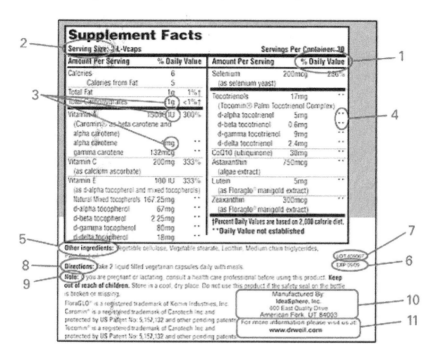

to pay attention to the serving size. Make sure you know how many to take. Some labels actually say take four. If you are watching your weight, you may have to consider the number of calories. Make sure the products have all the nutrients your body needs. Check the other ingredients and look up the words you do not know. Be sure to follow the directions. Notice and consider all the warning on the label. Be sure to keep your label. You never know, the product can be recalled. I usually take a picture and store all my medicines in an album—not for this reason alone, but in case of an emergency and to share with my doctors. Most current labels include a web address. Be sure to contact the company if any issues transpire.

Optional: only included for your practice of reading labels. Not meant to try to get you to drop your current regiment. Created just for your learning experience.

VENN DIAGRAM

Different   **Same**   **Different**

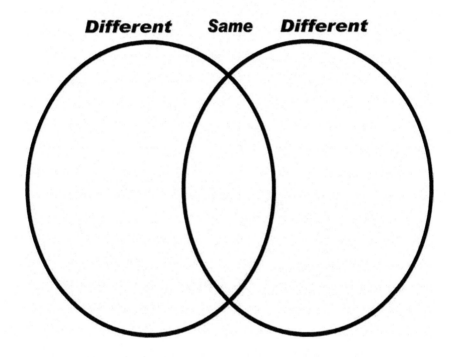

Alternative Classroom Activities and Directions:

Key chain with essential oil usage guide:

Simply cut out or tear out each shape. Use a whole puncher and punch one corner. Laminate if desired, and connect on a key ring.

Psalm 23 bookmarks and picture art:
Simply cut out the shape. Add embellishments and yarn.

For the picture frame, purchase a wood frame, add desired buttons, pot tabs, beads, etc., and cut Psalm 23 out for the frame.

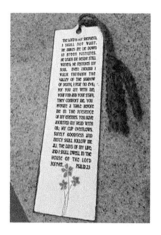
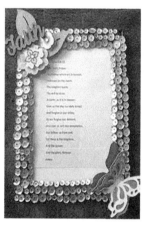

Oil-0 Game:
As the class is presented, the students cover their cards as the words are stated. Fill the oil-o card completely. Offer a gift to the winner. The author recommends this game to be used for review.

Construct your own essential oil Blends:
Below are a few steps to consider:

1. Determine the purpose of your blend (sleep, congestion, calming, anxiety).

2. Research oils that help with your specific need (example, peppermint is great for waking up and you would not want to use it in a calming blend).

3. Add your oils to a roller-bottle. Add a carrier oil halfway, then add your drops of oil and then fill the bottle the rest of the way with a carrier oil such as fractionated coconut oil.

Recipe station:

You may use these in any class that you are introducing the essential oil in.

Learning Center Method—If you choose to perform more than one at a time, I suggest using the puzzle method and having guests into groups, according to color or Bible chapter.

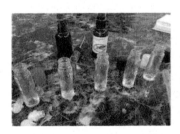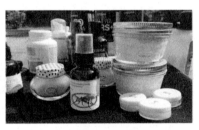

1. *Joseph's Dream Catcher /Roller-Ball Formula*
One .5 roller-ball set
Ten drops of juniper, bergamot, sandalwood, and black pepper essential oils
This mixture will help protect you from evil dreams while you sleep.

Joseph's Dream-Catcher Formula

2. *Roller-Ball Recipe for Joyfulness*
Five-milliliter bottle
Four drops of the following: citrus, orange, and grapefruit
Fill the rest of the bottle with distilled water or coconut oil.

3. *Heavy-Eyed Roller-Ball Remedy*
Five milliliters
Eight drops of Roman chamomile, 0 drops of bergamot, twelve drops
of frankincense
8 drops of bergamot.

4. *Influenza Bomb Remedy*
Five milliliters
Ten oreganos, twenty lemons, fifteen drops of protective blend
Fill halfway with fractionated coconut oil.

5. *Concentration Blend*
Twenty drops of wild orange, twenty drops of peppermint
Fill halfway with fractionated coconut oil.

6. *Wound Blend*
Fifteen drops of lavender, fifteen drops of melaleuca, ten drops of
fractionated coconut oil.

7. *Stuffy Schnozzle*
Twenty drops of respiratory blend, twelve drops of lime
Fill halfway with coconut oil.

8. *Cough Blend*
Twenty drops of respiratory blend, twelve drops of frankincense, and
half with fractionated coconut oil.

9. *Contusion Blend*
Ten drops of lavender, ten droplets of cypress, ten droplets of
frankincense
Ten droplets of fractionated coconut oil

10. *Tummy Blend*
Twenty droplets of wild orange and digestive blend
Fill halfway with fractionated coconut oil.

11. *Allergy Bomb*
Ten droplets of lemon, peppermint, lavender
Fill halfway with fractionated coconut oil.

12. *Stimulant Blend*
Fifteen drops of lemon, four drops of eucalyptus, three drops of peppermint, one drop of cinnamon

13. *Enhanced Memory*
Ten drops of lavender, eight drops of lemon, five drops of rosemary, and one drop of cinnamon

14. *ADHA Liquid Relief*
drops of lavender, thirty-five drops of valor, thirty drops of stress blend, fifteen drops of patchouli, forty drops of carrier oil
Put in a fifteen-milliliter bottle; add aroma glide top.
Apply to feet and wrists as needed. On the next few pages are images that you can create a key-chain charm ring. Copy and cut-out the images. Then, tape both sides of the hexagons because this will make them more durable. Next, whole punch, and add the shapes to the key chain.

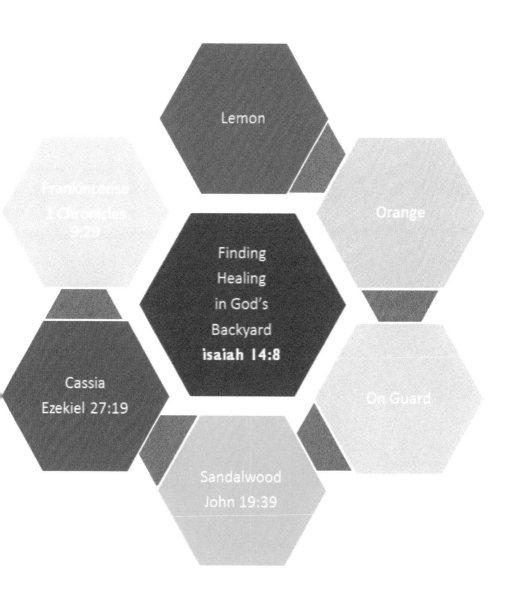

Lemon

Frankincense
1 Chronicles
9:29

Orange

Finding
Healing
in God's
Backyard
isaiah 14:8

Cassia
Ezekiel 27:19

On Guard

Sandalwood
John 19:39

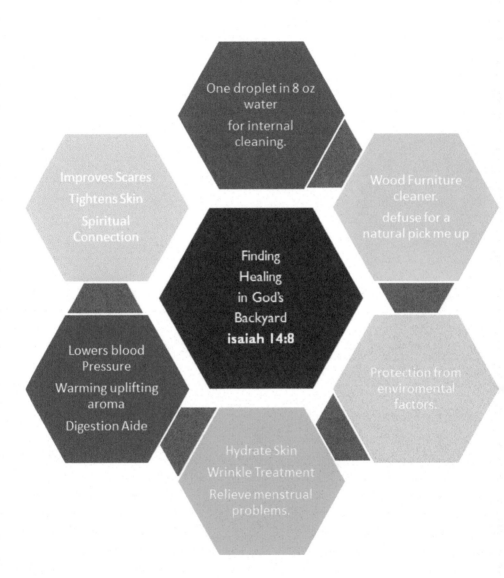

One droplet in 8 oz water

for internal cleaning.

Improves Scares

Tightens Skin

Spiritual Connection

Wood Furniture cleaner.

defuse for a natural pick me up

Finding Healing in God's Backyard **isaiah 14:8**

Lowers blood Pressure

Warming uplifting aroma

Digestion Aide

Protection from enviromental factors.

Hydrate Skin

Wrinkle Treatment

Relieve menstrual problems.

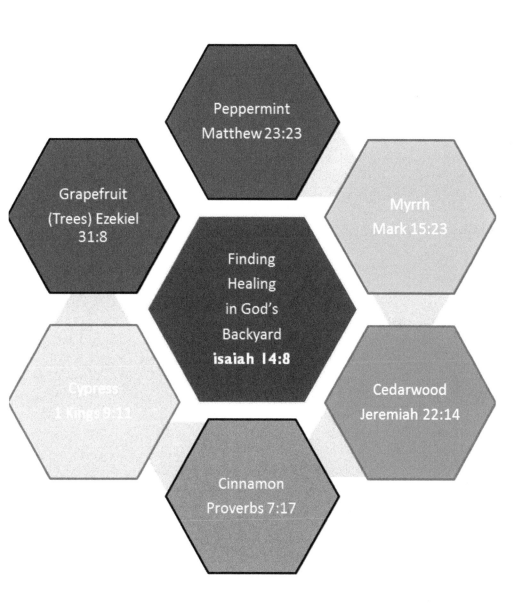

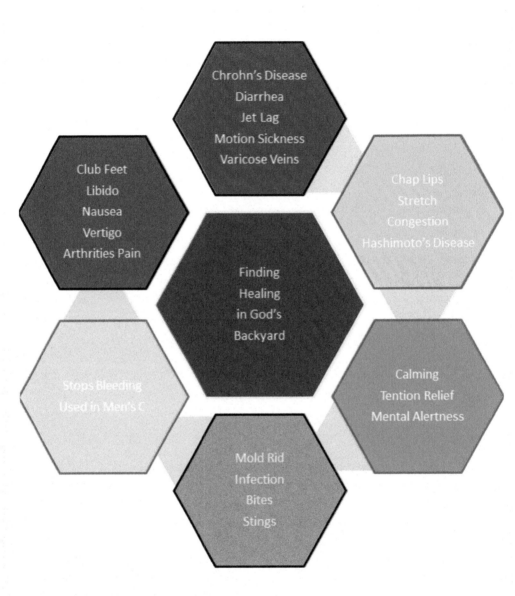

Oil -O Card

O   I   L   -   O

Word List:

Cedarwood Bible Cinnamon Snack Frankincense
Christ Myrrh Aloes Mint Spices Perfume Modern
Anointed Biblical essential oil Sweet Savors Incense

Healthy uses Altar Embalming Serve odors aromatherapy Amen Proverbs Genesis 1 Peter Ecclesiastes 1 Corinthians Exodus James Matthew John Paul Jews Hebrews Relief Aid Balm Body Soul Mind Benefits sickness Shepherd sheep joy definition scripture verse emotion smell odor God Father immortally read Please surrender redeemed repent cleanse soul bitter teardrop Prayer manages Physicians life womb Class Jesus give help

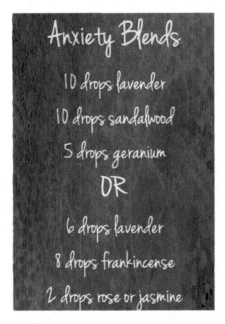

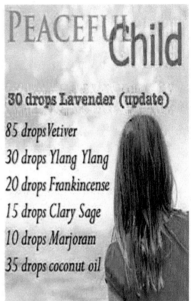

Home- Made Non-Toxic Cleaners

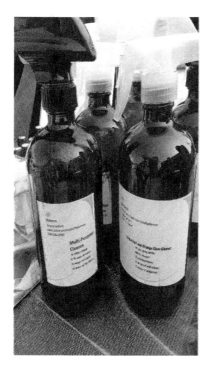
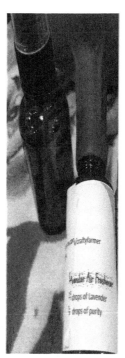

About the Author

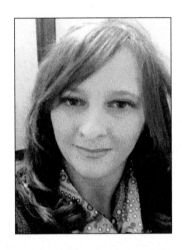

Jessica Linhart is a wife and mother of three. She was a special education teacher (MA degree+), but due to her medical conditions, she had to resign. Her family resides on a small family farm in Elkview, West Virginia. She is a great ponder and enthusiastic speaker in small-group ministry and in the classroom. She teaches Sunday school and is the director of food ministries at Silas Gospel Tabernacle, in Charleston West Virginia. Jessica is passionate about finding ways to reach people. In this book, she identifies God's medicine (essential oils), explains the use of essential oils in accordance with biblical meanings, and offers recipes for today's world. She understands the United States medical field and wants to seek those who are locate and those who don't know Christ before he returns.

May The Holy Spirit guide your study!

Jessica Linhart

CPSIA information can be obtained
at www.ICGtesting.com
Printed in the USA
FSOW03n0812310317
32392FS

9 781635 751185